When
Color
Fades

When Color Fades

a novel by C.J. Clark

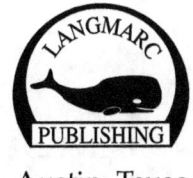

LANGMARC
PUBLISHING

Austin, Texas

WHEN COLOR FADES
A NOVEL BY C.J. CLARK

Cover Artist: C.J. Clark
Cover layout: Michael Qualben
Back cover photo by Rudy Ximenez Photography
RSX Digital Images • rximenez.tripod.com

Published by LangMarc Publishing
P.O. 90488
Austin, TX 78709
www.langmarc.com
langmarc@booksails.com

ISBN: 1-880292-41-6 • 978-1880292-419
Library of Congress Control Number: 2011923409

Dedicated to the memory
of my great aunt,
Lillian Nattier

'Because these wings are no longer wings to fly
But merely vans to beat the air
The air which is now thoroughly small and dry
Smaller and dryer than the will
Teach us to care and not to care
Teach us to sit still.'

T.S. Eliot
Ash Wednesday
1930

"Year that trembled and reel'd beneath me!
Your summer wind was warm enough,
Yet the air I breathed froze me"
— Walt Whitman

CHAPTER 1

Annabelle

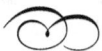

Annabelle Storm stepped out of her car to inspect the damage. She tucked wisps of graying hair behind her ears, pressing her fingertips into her temples. She'd driven her husband's car off the highway into a blue-bonnet meadow leaving a path of smashed flowers in her wake. She stared at the wildflowers. She couldn't remember doing anything like this before. It wasn't truly an accident, but she did have a flat tire. She kicked at the tire, scuffing her church shoes as though this would somehow help.

She had lost her way. That was it. It had dawned on her that she had lost her direction and in a flash of panic, she'd jerked her husband's Honda off the road, causing the tire to blow out. It could have happened to anyone. She hadn't even driven that far. Wasn't she just on her way to church? She glanced down at her rose-colored dress, gray scarf and matching heels as if to confirm this.

Quite clearly she would have to call the Auto Club. She had a vague recollection of where she had been and where she was going, but everything in between seemed misplaced.

A sultry breeze swept across the spring meadow stirring wildflowers into a slow dance. When the breeze subsided, all became hushed as though the land held its breath. Nothing moved. Ancient oaks reached gnarled arms to the earth, not quite touching. The blue wash of the Texas sky paled in contrast to the richly-colored blue-bonnets growing wild along the ranch road that sliced through uninhabited country. It was Sunday. A good day for a scenic drive for anyone in search of wildflowers. But no one came. No onlookers. No cars. Nothing. Only the sound of a crow cawing in the far distance.

A buzzard circled low in the sky. The day was warm and muggy, a prelude to summer. Annabelle loosened the scarf around her neck. Beads of sweat formed on her upper lip. She reached into her purse for her billfold. The Auto Club card was buried under business cards with scribbled phone numbers and addresses. She felt as though she was looking through someone else's purse. Why had she kept all these cards? Hadn't it been a while now since her husband had retired? She'd spent so much time alone lately, she wasn't certain. She reached for her cell phone, put on her glasses, then slowly jabbed at the buttons, dialing the Auto Club.

"Hello?" she said, "Yes, uh, my name is Mrs. Stanley Storm. I will need some assistance. I've had a flat tire." She listened intently to the reply.

"Well, yes, that's the thing. My husband usually— I'm a bit lost, you see. I don't see any signs, but I know I'm on the ranch road out of south Austin traveling east from Wintergray Ranch to Shepherd's Methodist Church." She stopped, again listening to the reply. She read the numbers of her Auto Club membership into the phone.

"Yes, yes that sounds right. I'm traveling east, I think." She shielded her eyes with her free hand and gazed up at the sky, noticing that the buzzard had been joined by two more buzzards that now circled above a stand of prickly pear cactus. She blotted her upper lip with the hem of her scarf.

"Thirty minutes? Well yes. I'm supposed to be at church—I think." She hung up and sank into the front seat of her car. She began to thumb through the contents of her purse. Other than her driver's license, there were two photos. One was a photo taken with her husband Stanley. It was taken twenty years earlier, and she marveled at how solid they looked with their perfect smiles and crisp clothes.

The wave of grief that washed over her as she thought of Stanley began to mount into panic. Stanley had left her. He was dead. Had it been a few weeks ago or had a whole month passed? Or had it been only days since he'd been fatally struck by the car of a drunken teenager who shot through a red light? The boy had plowed into Stanley's pick-up truck and never looked back.

The other photo was of her daughter Lily as a toddler. Annabelle felt a surge of protectiveness followed by disapproval as she stared at the photo. It was just that Lily reminded Annabelle so much of herself as a child. Bright, but naïve. Attractive, but ordinary. Now Lily was in the world living her life, making her own mistakes. The truth was that no matter how hard she'd tried over the years, Annabelle could not look at her daughter without feeling a spark of fresh misery well up from her own past. Her relationship with her daughter had turned hostile, even explosive. Now they were irreversibly detached from each other. She had no idea how to reach out to Lily.

Annabelle took a deep breath, held it, then slowly exhaled, making a small whistling noise. She missed

Stanley so much that sometimes it hurt to breathe. She rested her head against the back of the car seat and closed her eyes until sleep began to envelop her like a soft blanket.

The rumble of an approaching wrecker startled her awake. She rubbed furiously at her eyes, knocking her glasses to the floor of the car. She stepped out onto the road to flag down the driver. A car sped by from the opposite direction, slowing as it passed her. Children in the back seat gaped and pointed at her. She quickly looked away.

"Had some trouble finding you, ma'am," the burly driver said in a booming voice as he stopped beside Annabelle. His arm dangled out the open window revealing a tattoo of a crucifix on his forearm and tobacco-yellowed fingernails. Annabelle held her breath against the stench of exhaust fumes mixed with stale beer. The driver was snapping chewing gum and grinning. "So, what happened? Run off the road?"

"Yes. That is more or less the situation," Annabelle shouted, trying to be heard over the roar of the wrecker. She wrapped her arms across her waist, backing away as the driver stepped out of the cab and ambled over to the flat tire. The man had huge plump hands and to Annabelle, it seemed the man would have trouble gripping any sort of tool.

"Well, lets see. I don't think you're gonna need to be towed out of here. The ground is pretty level. No ditch. You oughta be able to back right out and be on your way. Maybe even make it to church. You'll be late, but you should make it for the benediction anyway." The driver glanced from the car to Annabelle, then settled his gaze on the flat tire. He'd taken off his baseball cap to smooth strands of thinning hair. His manner was jovial and inviting. He turned back to Annabelle and eyed her with open curiosity. A long uncomfortable moment passed. When Annabelle made no attempt at conversation, the driver shrugged, then retrieved the spare tire from the trunk.

Annabelle stood, unmoving. She felt incapable and embarrassed. She desperately missed her husband. It had always been Stanley's belief that when one felt inadequate in any situation that it was best to remain silent. Disarm them with silence, he had always said. He'd taught Annabelle how to change a flat tire but she was, after all, in her church clothes. She thumbed through her purse again, pretending she was searching for something. Something. Anything. A folded paper fell to the ground. She picked it up and opened it.

It was a letter Stanley had written, with a business card tucked inside. She looked at it as though seeing it for the first time but was gradually seized with a blurred but powerful memory. Dread began to overcome her. On the front of the business card was the inscription of a neurologist in Austin. Annabelle suddenly remembered the man clearly. The neurologist had been a small studious man with dark curly hair who spoke carefully and watched her over the rim of his glasses. His eyes had been a soft brown and very kind. He'd actually sat beside Annabelle and talked with her as one would to an old friend. Annabelle had been resistant to the doctor's words. She remembered that now. She remembered that the doctor had asked Stanley if there was anyone he would want him to call. Family. Friends. Anyone? Stanley had said no. There was no one.

Annabelle turned the card over. On the back, were the tiny scribbled notes she had made while the doctor was talking to her. *Mrs. Storm, you have Alzheimer's. An insidious disease. No cure. Only gets worse. No cure. Insidious, insidious, insidious...no cure, insidious...* Insidious. She had written the word *insidious* several more times until she had run out of room on the card.

Annabelle looked at the letter. It was one of several Stanley had started writing to their daughter after they'd returned home. After they'd shared a bottle of their favorite red wine. After they'd sat limply on their back terrace watching the sun set orange behind the emerald hills. After they had cried soundless tears. It had been just another sunset except that everything had changed. Their world had been altered. No, it was shattered. They had worked so hard over the years only to face this ending. She wasn't sure if Stanley had even intended to send the letter to Lily. He had never wanted to alarm her. Now Lily would never know. Annabelle opened it, unfolding the paper carefully and read the words, which now seemed foreign.

Dear Lily,

You will only be reading these words in the event of my demise. I have asked your mother to give it to you. Above all, I have not wanted to burden you with this, but here it is.

The neurologist has just informed us that Annabelle has early onset Alzheimer's disease. Although I do not want to believe this, the tests have confirmed it to be true. I am now trying to arrange things so that life will be easier for your mother. She will need to stop driving soon. She will need constant supervision at home. She's so young—younger than I am—it just doesn't seem possible. I think you know your mother has behaved a bit unpredictably for some time. I have known something was wrong for the last several years, but I refused to acknowledge it.

I know you and your mother have your differences. And I know that those differences have caused you two to become hopelessly alienated over the years. I wish I could reveal things to you that might make you understand your mother better. There are things you will never know unless Annabelle chooses to tell you. Your mother has always loved you dearly. Just remember that, please.

You must rise above your estrangement and understand that when I am gone, she will need you desperately.

It is an insidious disease, Lily. I have no real courage as your mother and I begin this final journey together. I just want you to know that— —-

Annabelle stopped reading. The wrecker driver was staring at her. She quickly wadded the letter into a tight ball and jammed it into the bottom of her purse, knowing she would later destroy it.

"Yep. Well I'm done here. You can be on your way, ma'am," the driver said, wiping his hands on his pant legs. He watched Annabelle as though he was not sure what to do about her. "Ma'am, are you okay? You don't seem well."

"Yes, of course," Annabelle's voice faltered, then became defiant. "I am quite well." Did this wrecker driver have no manners? Why did he continue to gawk at her? She tucked her billfold into her purse and without looking up added quietly, "Well actually, I'm not certain where I am, to be honest. I'd like to go home now. I'm just off course a little bit."

"No problem. I can help you. What's the address?"

Instead of telling the driver the address, Annabelle pulled out her billfold again and thrust her driver's license toward him. The driver took it from her, looked at it, then raised his eyebrows slightly. Something in his manner shifted.

"Ma'am, is this your current address?" the driver finally asked.

"Well, yes, of course," Annabelle said, feeling more and more uncertain.

"Because this is only a mile from here at best. It's just over that hill." The driver pointed to the west, then looked quickly back at Annabelle.

"Are you absolutely sure?" Annabelle asked, incredulous, "because I believe you are wrong. I've been driving for quite some time this morning." She glanced at the Honda's gas gauge. It was on empty. How could she have used a whole tank of gas? She stared at the car keys in her hand. There were too many of them. Why were there so many keys?

"On your way to church," the driver said. His booming voice had softened.

"Yes, church. I was just going to church. Shepherd's United Methodist Church. It's a very large church." She tried to picture the church in her mind but couldn't. Church was just a word rolling off her tongue.

"Oh yes ma'am, I'm real familiar with it. It's only another few miles to the east. A straight shot. Yeah, but it's too late, the services are over now. Guess there's always next Sunday, eh?" The driver handed Annabelle's license back to her. "Say, why don't you follow me back to your house? You know– just in case there's a problem with the tire or something. I'm headed that direction anyway."

Annabelle knew this was a lie. She wanted to protest, to tell the driver that she'd made a mistake. Of course she knew where her home was. But instead she nodded, avoiding eye contact with the man.

It took only minutes for them to arrive at Annabelle's house. The relief she felt at seeing her home flooded her with a deep sense of well-being. Here was her mansion nestled in the rolling hills. Here was her own private world, surrounded by live oaks and walkways bordered with extensive flower beds of sage, lantana, Spanish lavender, red cannas, orange lilies, and deep purple irises that now greeted and accepted her.

Annabelle suppressed the urge to kick off her shoes and bolt to the house. She glanced back at the wrecker driver who waved at her uncertainly but did not pull away from the curb. What was the man waiting for anyway? She walked briskly up the long winding path to the massive front porch with its matching rocking chairs that were rocking slightly in the spring breeze. No one had ever actually sat in these chairs sipping tea and discussing politics. No one had ever sat in these chairs, waiting for the mail to arrive or for grandchildren to come visit. So, it seemed the chairs sat empty, year after year, rocking themselves in quiet rebellion when the wind was just right. Annabelle fumbled with her keys. She could feel the eyes of the driver on her. She tried the door. To her amazement it was unlocked. Had she forgotten to lock the door? She dismissed this as an impossibility and stepped inside.

The foyer was cool and dark with its granite tile floor, high ceiling and slender, delicate windows that let in only the tiniest bit of light. She shut the door behind her and took a deep breath. Home. She was home, she was safe. The grandfather clock chimed from the study. Annabelle looked at her wristwatch. For a long time she stood, gathering her thoughts, wondering what she was supposed to be doing. She looked down at her rose-colored dress with the gray scarf and at her shoes. Her shoes were scuffed, but she decided the scuff marks were not all that noticeable. She glanced at her wristwatch again, then smoothed her hair into place. She would need to find Stanley. Wouldn't it be time to go to church soon?

*"Lady of silences
Calm and distressed
Torn and most whole
Rose of memory
Rose of forgetfulness"*
— *T.S. Eliot*

Chapter 2

Lily

Lily Storm ran as though she was being chased. She ran faster and faster until her breath came in short puffs and sweat trickled down her face. The sky above her was the bluest she had ever seen. It was a ceiling of blue, bearing down on her, making her want to run even quicker. Like a child she ran, slicing through the icy April air, her face reddened with wind burn. She could feel the numbness of it, but she kept on running down the middle of the old gravel road. A deer bolted across her path. She was surprised how much noise her running made. Her legs were heavy and her feet felt like big blobs of cement. But she kept racing onward, looking straight ahead at the endless road lined on either side with tall trees and thick underbrush. She was too out of shape to run like this. But she had to. She had to run away. Her feet became cumbersome and plodding.

She wanted to cry, but stopped herself. She would not cry. She had to be strong. Her breathing became more labored as she fought back tears. Her legs ached, pain shot through her calves. She looked down, willing her feet to quicken.

Suddenly she stopped. She stopped so quickly that she became dizzy and had to steady herself as she began to laugh. Her laughter filled the sky as she held her sides. What had she been thinking? She looked at her feet again. Hiking boots. She had been trying to run in her heavy-duty hiking boots.

For a moment she stood motionless, silent except for her breathing, which was still coming in gasps. Annabelle, she thought. It's because of Annabelle. Lily remembered storming out of the cabin into the chill because of their argument. And it had been so absurd, really. They'd argued over some red box or chest or whatever Annabelle said it was. She couldn't even picture it because each time Annabelle spoke of it, she described it differently. Once Annabelle said it was a large storage chest, then an old shoe box, then a red suitcase. Either way, Annabelle was obsessed with finding it.

Annabelle was so obsessed that she had insisted on having Lily drive her fifteen hundred miles away from their home in central Texas to their cabin in northwestern Minnesota at a time of year when crusts of snow were still melting into a hesitant green spring. They hadn't found it. Annabelle said it had important documents and letters she needed. That was all she would say. Important documents and letters. Then her voice would trail off as she drifted into some distant thought. Why do you need to find it right now, Lily had asked her. As usual, Annabelle waved Lily away and stared into the empty space ahead of her. It had always been that way, but since Lily's father had been killed in a car accident the month before, it was even worse. And there were other things.

Suddenly Lily spotted a moving cloud of brown dust on the road ahead of her and watched as a minivan came into view. It slowed as it came closer. Looking directly ahead, Lily held up her hand in an anonymous wave. She heard a protesting crunch of gravel beneath tires as the vehicle began to decelerate. Inwardly she winced, willing the minivan to drive on. It stopped beside her.

"Lily? Lily Storm!" A woman's voice bellowed from the minivan's open window.

Lily looked up to see the smiling face of her childhood friend, Tess Olson. She walked over to the driver's side just as Tess eagerly flung open the door. Lily had to jump back to avoid being struck.

"Oh my god, I am so sorry. Are you okay?" Tess hopped out of the minivan and laughed as she gave Lily a quick hug then stood back, openly surveying her. "Hey, are you sure you're okay? You look awful. No, no–I mean thin, really thin. Or exhausted. Or something. What is it?"

"I'm okay. I probably do look awful. You, on the other hand, look fabulous," Lily elongated the word fabulous with a forced southern drawl. Tess did look fabulous as always. Lily felt like a graceless clod next to her friend. At age thirty five, Tess was as trim and athletic as she'd been in high school. Her Scandinavian blonde hair was cropped into short chaotic curls. Her ice blue eyes were piercing. Tess's limitless energy might have irritated Lily if the two women hadn't grown up sharing their separate worlds like sisters.

They'd remained close despite the fact that since elementary school, they saw each other only during the summer months. Their lives had unfolded so differently. Tess's marriage to her high school boyfriend, Sam Olson, was rock solid. Their son Teddy was maturing into a promising young man. And yet, Lily was still bumbling her way through life never quite certain of anything.

"What are you doing up here, Lily? You never come up this early in the year. Is everything all right?" Tess paused, still studying her friend. "Oh wait—Lily, I am so, so sorry. It's your dad. I know you must be devastated."

"Yes, well—," Lily started, then stopped as she felt tears well up inside her.

"You were so close to your dad. I know this has to be so hard on you. Especially with you and Annabelle being so alienated all these years." There was sudden caution mixed with curiosity in Tess's voice, "So, how is Annabelle?"

"Yeah, well, you know Mom. What can I say? She's grief stricken of course, but what's so odd is how obsessed she's getting with the most unpredictable things."

"But you'd expect that, wouldn't you? Your mom and dad were totally inseparable," Tess said. Then watching Lily's expression darken added, "What is it? What do you mean exactly?"

Lily wasn't certain how to answer. It wasn't entirely clear to her. She just knew that her mother had fallen apart immediately after her dad died, but that just as quickly she had become stern and filled with purpose. Instead of embracing Lily in their mutual time of sadness, Annabelle began to pull away. Lily wondered if she would ever truly comprehend this person who was her mother. She felt intensely alone. Tess was the only person she could confide in about Annabelle's erratic demeanor.

"Hey, want to go into town and get some coffee? It's still early. Maybe we could get some of those carrot spice muffins at the Gray Dawn Café," Lily said, changing the subject. "We could talk. You know."

"Well, sure," Tess put on her sunglasses and flashed a toothpaste-white smile. "Hey, why not? Let's go."

Lily paused by the door of the van. For a split second, she considered going back to the cabin to tell Annabelle where she was going. But why? Why did she feel uneasy about leaving Annabelle alone? Annabelle wouldn't care. They would probably be gone only an hour, if even that.

An unexpected sense of buoyancy came over Lily. It suddenly didn't seem all that long ago that she was a teenager piling into Tess's old Ford Mustang at this very same spot. It had been one of those sweltering summer days, rare for this far north. They had kicked off their shoes, leaving them by the side of the road, then sped away like bank robbers fleeing the scene of a crime. Tess had rolled all the car windows down and turned the radio loud to some symphonic rock song. They made up their own lyrics, crooning along with the music, letting their long hair whip around in the wind.

Lily remembered that they were smoking cigarettes and that it didn't matter where they were going. It didn't matter that inelegant Lily Storm was riding around with perfect Tess Olson. Tess had just whisked them away, wildly turning down every washboard country road she came to.

Lily hadn't cared if she ever went home. She only knew that she'd argued viciously with Annabelle about something absurd. Her dad had taken Annabelle's side and Lily was furious. No, she'd been incredulous. Her dad had always either remained quiet or taken Lily's side. And Annabelle had always listened to him.

"Lily?" Tess eyed her friend with curiosity. "What is it? Did you change your mind?"

"No, no. I was just thinking about that time we left our shoes here on the road and drove all over the county like maniacs. You told me we were erasing the argument between Annabelle and me." Lily sighed, still locked into the memory. "It worked. Sort of."

"Our shoes? What? Oh good lord, that was ages ago." Suddenly laughing, Tess said, "Didn't we end up in the ditch? Oh yeah, that was trouble."

The two of them laughed like teenagers, briefly reliving their misadventure. But Lily's laughter faded when she caught a glimpse of herself in the minivan's side mirror. Tess was right. She did look awful. If she'd ever had looks, she'd lost them now. Her brown hair was pulled back tightly into a ponytail. She wore no make-up whatsoever, no attempt to hide the little lines around her brown eyes. She was so thin that her clothes hung on her like rags.

"I need a makeover."

"What? Where is this coming from? Did Annabelle tell you that? Okay. Yes, we do need to talk. Get in. Let's go," Tess said as Lily climbed into the minivan.

Lily noticed that Tess took the longest route to town. It was as though she knew that Lily needed the car ride even more than she needed coffee at the Gray Dawn. She felt her tension ease as she gazed out over the expanse of deep green meadows extending to the horizon on either side of them. Wisps of blanched clouds stretched across the powder blue sky. In the far distance a ghost-like formation of Canadian geese eased their way across the atmosphere. The geese were flying north to Canada with unwavering purpose.

Tess turned off the highway onto a narrow gravel road. The minivan lurched and objected as the road became winding and steep. After the first rise in the road, the rolling green meadows were replaced by vast birch woods. Bits of blue sky broke through shimmering green leaves, illuminating the stately white tree trunks. Lily rolled down her window and inhaled deeply. She'd always felt there was something spiritual about birch woods, something light and inviting.

"I miss this," Lily said. She did miss the rolling green meadows, the wide open spaces, the mystical wooded landscapes. She missed emerald greens, cobalt blues and Canadian geese that appeared out of nowhere. She missed being able to take in the entire expanse of sky with one sweeping glance. She missed having friends who didn't pass judgment.

"I know." Tess glanced briefly at Lily.

The Gray Dawn Café was nearly empty except for a few of the regulars sipping on coffee and scanning the Minneapolis Sunday paper even though it was already Tuesday. An overpowering scent of freshly brewed coffee and baked bread filled the café.

Lily and Tess slid into a booth next to a window overlooking the town's main street. Tess motioned to a man behind the coffee bar. He was wearing a long apron over faded blue jeans and a gray flannel shirt. His light blue eyes and blonde hair were almost the same as Tess's. He nodded at her, then slowly broke into a boyish grin. Tess smiled at him as he approached with his order pad.

"Hello, Tess. What can I get for you ladies?" He nodded at a customer entering the café, then looked back at Tess expectantly.

"Hi, Will. You remember Lily Storm?" Tess tipped her head in Lily's direction.

Will turned toward Lily, appraising her presence as though she had suddenly dropped from the ceiling. He raised his eyebrows momentarily, then settled into a warm smile. Lily shifted uneasily. She'd been infatuated with Will Larson as far back as she could remember. She felt foolish thinking of it now. She looked away.

"Well, yeah, of course. Lily. How are you then?" He had a strong Canadian accent. "Haven't seen you in a long time. Kind of early for you to be this far north, isn't it? We might still get some snow, ya know." He glanced out the window and squinted up at the sky, as though this might happen at any moment.

"Will is the new owner of the Gray Dawn," Tess interrupted. "He's done an unbelievable job fixing up the place." She turned back to Will and said, "Hey, do you think we could we have some coffee and carrot spice muffins?"

"Yeah, sure. I just ground some coffee beans. Coffee and muffins coming up." With that, he turned and disappeared behind the swinging doors leading into the kitchen.

"I think you made him nervous," Tess laughed. "He always liked you, Lily. Did you know his wife ran off with some musician a few years ago? All he has now is this café."

"Yeah, I think you told me, but for Pete's sake, Tess, I'm sure I didn't make him nervous. Will Larson barely remembers me." Lily was so certain of this that she suddenly felt a little sad. She was thirty-five years old, living her adult life, and yet she could still feel a little tug of an adolescent emotion.

"Lily, listen. About Annabelle. I don't get her, but I do love her in a way. You know that. But I just hate that whatever happened between you two has caused you to have such a low opinion of yourself. You are easily one of the most captivating people I have ever known. You are charming and you're brilliant. You are an absolutely beautiful person. Lily, are you even listening to me?"

Lily smiled vaguely but didn't answer. She looked out the window at an elderly woman shuffling along the sidewalk. The old woman seemed lost and uncertain, looking into the little shop windows. Finally the woman stopped, turned around, then hobbled into the post office just as a kid raced by on a skateboard.

"I'm surprised they let that kid skateboard on the sidewalk," Lily said finally. "Sometimes I wish I could do that. You know, skateboarding. I think I'd be good at it."

"Oh, okay so you're not listening." Tess sighed, "well, anyway, how's work?"

"Really good." Lily enjoyed talking about her job. "Who would have guessed that rescuing half dead plants would lead to owning my own garden shop one day?"

"I know! Remember you told me how you used to go into that awful garden center and buy all those half-priced plants that had been so badly neglected? Such empathy," Tess clicked her tongue.

"I don't know if it was empathy exactly. That stupid store manager just started giving me carts full of dead plants. I became oddly obsessed with it. It was a little crazy—driving away with all those wilted and crispy flowers. The only reason they were dying was because he put everything in the blazing sun and never watered. I didn't have room in my apartment for all those revived plants, so I'd have to take them back to the garden shop." She paused, then laughed. "Somehow it never seemed right, because I always wondered if the plants I was rescuing were the same plants I'd returned a few weeks before. Annabelle thought the whole thing was beneath me."

"Well, yeah, Annabelle always did have pretty high expectations of you."

Glancing again out the window, Lily noticed the elderly woman coming out of the post office carrying a large parcel. She was struggling against the weight of it. An older man walked up to her and took the package. They stood talking for a moment, then slowly began to make their way down the sidewalk just as the skateboarding kid narrowly missed them from behind. Lily imagined skateboarding alongside the boy, racing ahead of him, telling him to eat her dust.

"Dangerous kid," Lily said as she folded her hands on the table and smiled at Tess. "Anyway, pretty amazing stroke of luck that I was able to buy that garden shop. I had no real qualifications. I'd always figured on being a journalist." She shrugged, then added, "So, how are Sam and Teddy?"

Before Tess had a chance to respond, Will Larson returned with a pot of steaming coffee and a tray of muffins. Lily inhaled the spicy aroma of freshly baked carrot muffins and rich dark coffee. She watched Will as he poured coffee into their ceramic mugs. He didn't seem the least bit nervous to her.

"So Lily, how long are you up here for then?" Will dragged a chair over to the table and dropped into it sideways, dangling his arms across the back. Lily had his full attention.

"We probably won't be here even a week. I brought Mom so she could find some box with documents in it. She's pretty intent on finding it." Lily stirred her coffee, watching white cream swirl into the black liquid, lightening it to beige.

"Sorry about your dad's accident," Will said. "He was a good guy."

"Thanks—" Lily took her coffee mug in both hands and sipped, closing her eyes.

The phone rang from behind the bar. Will jumped up, signaling the end of their conversation. He became absorbed in the phone call. Lily watched him for a moment, then looked at Tess who was also watching Will.

"Are you still writing poetry?" Tess asked, turning back to Lily. She spread butter onto her carrot muffin, watched it melt, then took a small bite.

"I could paper my bedroom wall with the stuff I've written." Lily sighed as she surveyed the interior of the café. The floors were red brick and the walls were knotty pine. There were several surrealistic paintings on the walls. "This café looks a lot different than it used to. Who did all these paintings? They're very um—unusual."

"Teddy."

"Your son, Teddy? I didn't know he could paint. I thought he was off at the university majoring in forest management or something." Lily studied the paintings appreciatively.

"He was, but Ted's – taking a break – to find himself." Tess shuddered visibly. She began to search through her handbag and pulled out a folded napkin. "Remember this?" She produced a tattered napkin and read the inscribed words aloud, "*Wasn't this once called the Skogmo Café? We laugh lightly, because neither of us can really say. We order broth and chowder, and drink the soup of our separate winters. Of your life, made of solid things, and of mine, made of tiny single splinters.*"

"You kept that?" Lily laughed. "It's kind of good in a terrible way."

"What does that mean exactly? I love your poetry. I fully expect you to become Poet Laureate of the United States someday. You'll win the Pulitzer, of course. You'll hobnob with all the other great contemporary poets, you know, T.S. Eliot, Dylan Thomas, E.E. Cummings...."

"Tess, they're all dead."

"Oh, yeah. Well, anyway, you'll invite me to tea from time to time at your studio villa in Cornwall and read me all of your latest work," Tess said.

"Cornwall?"

"Well, okay. What about Greece or Hawaii or New Mexico or New Zealand?"

The two women laughed. Will looked in their direction and smiled. A delivery truck driver with a clipboard was talking to him. The phone rang again.

"Gray Dawn," Will answered the phone as he signed papers, then handed the clipboard back to the delivery driver. "Sure, Tess is right here. Are you okay?" There was a pause, then," Uh-huh, uh-huh. Are you sure? Where exactly? Uh-huh. Well, who is she? Man, that's pretty weird." He glanced over at Lily, then looked away quickly. "No, wait. I'm telling you she's right here. Well, okay. I'll tell her." He hung up and stared at the phone, his hand still on the receiver.

"Will?" Tess stood up. "What's wrong? Who was that?"

"It was Teddy." Will looked first at Lily, then Tess. "There's a problem at the farm."

"What kind of problem?" Tess asked warily.

"I don't know, Tess. It's strange." He turned to Lily and said, "Yeah, I think your mom may be out there at the farm. She's down by the lake on the dock. Something's not right about her, Lily."

"What do you mean? Farm? What farm?" Lily jumped to her feet, knocking over her coffee mug. A puddle of coffee spilled over the edge of the table and trickled to the floor.

"It's Sam's dad's farm. Teddy's been staying out there this spring," Tess said as she grabbed a napkin and started mopping up coffee. "The property backs up to the lake. But I wonder how Annabelle got out there. Why is she on the dock? Will, tell me exactly what Teddy said."

"He said that she just showed up. He could see her from the upstairs window. Didn't know who she was at first. When he went out to see if she needed help, she told him her husband had gone out in the boat and she was waiting for him to come back. He thought the whole thing was weird because she had no sweater, no jacket. And she's wearing no shoes, just socks. He brought her a thermos of hot tea because she was shivering so badly. The wind is freezing out there. But she won't leave. She's determined."

Lily slumped back into her chair and groaned. Annabelle had never done anything like this before. She put her head in her hands and sighed heavily.

"Well, we have to go. We have to go—now. C'mon Lily. What do you think is wrong with her?" Tess yanked

Lily to her feet. "Do you think she's just so overcome with grief that—"

"No, no. I don't know. Maybe that's it. Annabelle has been acting differently for several weeks now. Mostly just things she says, you know." Lily let herself be pulled along by Tess to the door of the Gray Dawn. She looked back at Will who nodded somberly.

"Is Teddy with her now?" Tess asked Will as she opened the door and pushed Lily out.

"Yeah, he went inside the house to call, that's all. She's standing at the edge of the dock. The water's really deep down at that end of the lake. Somebody needs to get her in. He said she looks frail and unsteady. Look, I can close up and drive you."

"No! No, please. It's okay. We can do this," Lily said emphatically, halfway out the door. The last thing she wanted was a dramatic scene.

The things she had hoped to discuss with Tess escaped her as they tore down gravel roads towards the farm. Tess seemed to know every back road in the county. Lily glanced at her. Tess's face was grim and determined. It was almost as though she had guessed what Lily had been going through. Maybe they didn't need to talk. The whole topic was so baffling anyway. Annabelle had memory lapses and at times seemed to forget how to complete the simplest tasks.

She'd always been critical and strict, but now Annabelle was prone to violent outbursts. Until recently, her strictness had come across as a sort of quiet firmness. It had been annoying, but never frightening. But now, Annabelle's behavior had begun to alarm Lily.

"You have to be the parent now," Tess said softly, as if reading Lily's thoughts.

Lily nodded, afraid if she spoke she might begin to cry and not stop.

Tess halted the minivan at a stop sign, startling a red-tailed hawk perched on a nearby fence post. The hawk stretched his wings as if contemplating flight. Lily remembered her father once telling her about a Native American belief of how a soaring hawk symbolizes a spirit set free. Her father had been such a kind, spiritual man. He had always provided a buffer between Lily and her mother, always explaining to Lily that her mother only wanted what was best for her.

Only weeks before his death, Lily's father had taken her hands in his and in a voice weary with repetition, he told her again to be patient with Annabelle, that there were reasons for her unyielding rigidity. Reasons that only Annabelle could reveal. And in time, perhaps Annabelle would. But, he told her, even if she chose not to, Lily needed to know that her mother's love for her had always been immeasurable.

Lily watched the red-tailed hawk lift off, soar away, hover, land on another fence post, then lift off to soar again. She was captivated by the hawk's low circling against the sapphire sky. It was hypnotic. The minivan lurched forward as they crossed a blacktop road and entered a narrow, rough lane. Lily's view of the hawk became obstructed by tall deciduous woods on either side of the van. They turned at a row of mailboxes onto another lane so overgrown that the grass underneath the van made a brushing sound as they drove.

"Watch out!" Lily suddenly shrieked, just as a dark form bolted across the road in front of them, causing Tess to slam on the brakes. "What in the—? It's Annabelle's dog! It's Caesar."

Lily flung open the door and bolted out of the van just as it halted. She chased after the dog. Rushing headlong into the woods, she tripped over fallen trees and underbrush, calling the dog's name. She fell face first into a pile of brush and sat, still shouting for the dog.

Finally the old basset hound stopped. He tilted his head to one side, looking at her. He had blood on his chest from what appeared to be a puncture wound and he was covered in soot. After a moment of uncertainty, he bounded over to her, clearly elated to see her. Lily hugged him then began to examine his wound.

"Good lord, was he shot? What do you think happened to him?" Tess said breathlessly as she ran up behind them. "Do you think he followed Annabelle?"

"I guess. But this is so far from the cabin. What is it? A mile? Two miles? I think he must have gotten into some barbed wire or something. You poor old guy. C'mon buddy let's get you home." Lily dabbed at his wound with a scarf Tess handed to her. Together they walked the dog back to the van. Neither of them spoke.

When they arrived at the farmhouse, Teddy met them in the driveway. Lily was amazed at how much he resembled Tess's husband Sam with his thick brown hair and deep blue eyes. But his demeanor was entirely different. Teddy's hair was long and tied back into a ponytail, causing him to appear delicate and much younger than his eighteen years. He seemed anxious and distraught.

"Hi Mom. Hi Lily. She's over there on the dock," he said turning to point to the lake. A strong cold breeze began to stir the treetops. Teddy folded his arms tightly across his chest and shivered a little. He was wearing paint-splattered jeans and a Minnesota State Parks T-shirt. "You can't really see her from here because of the bank. It's real steep. You better hurry. There's a strong north wind coming in. She's out there waiting for her husband."

"Teddy, her husband, Mr. Storm, he died just recently," Tess told her son as the three of them started for the lake.

"Oh, wow. I'm really sorry," Teddy said to Lily, then turning back to Tess he added, "But that's weird. Why does she think he's gone out in the boat? Doesn't she understand that—." He stopped abruptly when Tess shook her head at him.

A bank of violet clouds was rolling in from the north. The wind was beginning to blow in icy gusts off the lake. Lily wondered if Will might be right about a spring snowfall. Whitecaps crashed into shore and sloshed up onto the dock where Annabelle stood.

And there she was. Standing in her stocking feet at the very edge of the dock shielding her eyes with her hands, gazing out at the expanse of dark choppy water. There was a small thermos on the dock next to her. Her clothes and hair were being whipped around by the blustering wind. An eerie yellow light reflected off the water outlining her small frame, causing her to look like some sort of apparition. For one split second, Lily recalled a photograph she'd seen of her mother as a young woman standing just like this, on the edge of a dock with wind gusts threatening to toss her into the water. In the photo, her mother had one hand on her hip and the other shielding her eyes, scanning the horizon. Searching, searching. For what? Lily had often wondered what it was her mother was looking for and why she stood so close to the edge. It was a candid photo. Something someone had captured of her when she wasn't aware.

All of a sudden, Annabelle tipped forward, swayed slightly then righted herself. Lily sucked in a sharp breath and began to sprint towards her mother.

"Mom? What are you doing out here?" Lily was cautious as she got closer, afraid she might startle her mother, throwing her off balance.

When Annabelle didn't answer, Lily yelled louder against the wind, "Mom! You're too close to the edge. What are you doing out there? Can't you hear me?"

Annabelle turned to look at Lily who had just stepped onto the dock. Her face was drawn and sad. Lily thought she looked as though she'd been crying. Instead of answering, Annabelle held out her hand to wave. Or so Lily thought at first. The wave turned out to more of an attempt to motion Lily away as Annabelle turned back to stare out over the water.

"I'm not deaf, Lily. I heard you." Although she was shouting, Annabelle's voice was nearly lost in the sound of waves slamming into shore. She turned again to look at Lily who was on the dock walking slowly toward her. "Don't come any closer. I mean it. I'm waiting for your father. He's out in the boat. Left this morning. Should be back pretty soon." The gusting wind tore strands of hair away from her long gray braid, slapping them across her face. Annabelle didn't seem to notice.

"Mom!" Lily stepped closer as Annabelle turned back to the lake. "Dad's gone," she said, her voice still loud but gentle and cautious. "He passed away last month, don't you remember?"

Annabelle wheeled around, facing Lily. She took a menacing step forward, her face hot with anger. Lily instinctively moved back as though her mother had suddenly become a vicious predator. At that moment Lily didn't see Annabelle as frail or weak. She could only feel her mother's wrath spinning out of control.

"Why would you say such a hateful thing, Lily? What is the matter with you?" Annabelle's fury erupted into involuntary tremors. "How could you be so cruel?" She stepped back to the edge of the dock and began to scream out over the water, "Stanley! Stanley!"

"Mother, stop it! This is dangerous. Dad isn't out there." Lily moved swiftly towards Annabelle. She grabbed her arm but Annabelle jerked free, lost her balance then fell to her knees. The thermos Teddy had brought her earlier was hurled into the lake, disappearing into the swirl of black water.

"Leave me alone! I'm waiting for Stanley. Get away from me!" Annabelle was struggling to push Lily away and get to her feet. She was sobbing, trying to gain control. Finally she let Lily help her stand. "Stanley has gone out in the boat. I'm not leaving here." Her voice became a low hiss.

"Mom, it's okay. But Dad is gone. He didn't go out in the boat. Mother, Dad is—" Lily stopped short as she watched Annabelle become tense and resolute, her expression contorted between worry and rage.

Lily looked back at Tess and Teddy helplessly. They stood bewildered and unmoving on the shore. Teddy was visibly shivering now as the wind spit bone-chilling raindrops to the earth. Tess stepped onto the dock and began walking quickly toward Lily and Annabelle.

"Who's that?" Annabelle shielded her eyes, straining to recognize the person coming toward them. "Oh, is that you, Tess Olson? Goodness, what are you doing here?"

"Hello, Annabelle." Tess wasn't sure what to say. She and Lily exchanged apprehensive glances. "Well, I've come to see you, Annabelle. How about coming inside so we can visit? It is just freezing out here. The weather's taking a bad turn." She was trying to sound light and conversational, but Annabelle regarded her with sudden suspicion.

"No, no I can't. I'm waiting for Stanley to return. He went out in the boat this morning. I'm sure you understand." Annabelle's response was polite but her manner was cold. Suddenly she looked past Tess and pointed at Teddy who still stood on the shore. "That young man has been helping me. He knows about Stanley."

Lily and Tess turned to look at Teddy who stared back at them wide eyed. The roaring waves and high wind had only allowed him to hear part of their conversation. When he saw Annabelle smile at him, he waved at her uncertainly. She waved back as though she were waving at an old friend. Reluctantly he stepped onto the dock and moved toward them. All three women looked at him expectantly.

"Hello Mrs. Storm," Teddy said in a tentative voice just loud enough to be heard over the wind and waves. "I just spoke with Mr. Storm on the phone. He said he docked the boat in town and will be driving over here later after the bad weather passes."

His tone was so sincere and convincing. Lily marveled at his delivery of such a brazen lie. He locked eyes with Annabelle and would not look at Tess who gawked at him. He held out his hand to Annabelle, waiting.

"Oh." Annabelle seemed perplexed. A slow minute passed. Spitting rain turned to steady drops. The wind swirled around them. Annabelle began to rub her bare arms. She appeared to be considering Teddy's words. She frowned, bit her lip, then smiled. "Are you sure about this? You spoke with my husband? You spoke with Stanley?"

"Yes. Yes, I sure did," Teddy lied. He took another step towards her. She hesitated, then took his outstretched hand. He turned and led her off the dock. She trundled along behind him like a child in her damp socks, windswept hair and tattered clothes. Both Annabelle and Teddy were under dressed for the cold spring rain. Determined and purposeful, they marched on, leaving Lily and Tess gaping after them.

"Lily—" Tess began.

"So, you see? Do you see, Tess?" Lily felt tears sting her eyes. "I have never known my mother well, but this, this is not my mother."

They drove back to the cabin in silence. It was as though their reality had been altered into something intangible. Every so often Lily noticed Tess glance in the rearview mirror at Annabelle. Lily watched Annabelle in the side mirror as she patted her beloved basset hound, Caesar, who sat on the seat next to her. Annabelle seemed so small and defeated. She had never once questioned why her dog had a puncture wound to his chest.

Annabelle had no real recollection of walking the mile and a half to Teddy's grandfather's property. She didn't mention her husband or the boat. It didn't even seem to bother her when they'd left Teddy behind. She'd just waved and thanked him for his assistance, then mumbled something about what a nice boy he was. Even when Lily told her that he was Tess's son, Annabelle just nodded and commented about how he had grown into such a handsome young man.

The weather change had caused a chill to descend on the cabin. When they returned, Lily started a fire in the wood stove while Annabelle sat wrapped in blankets. Tess had stayed long enough to see that Annabelle was calm, then gave Lily a knowing look and mouthed the words, *call me* on her way out the door. Lily had decided not to say anything to her mother about the incident, partly because she had no idea what to say. Was she supposed to scold Annabelle for her irrational behavior? Or was she supposed to sit with her and gently remind her of her husband's accidental death a month before?

Lily felt lost without her father. He would have smoothed everything over. He would have been able to manage Annabelle. In fact, Lily wondered if he had been privately dealing with Annabelle's odd behavior for some time. There had always been a sort of secrecy between her parents. Even as a child, Lily could remember the two of them cutting short their hushed conversations when she entered the room. It had only begun to bother her when she reached high school age. She'd always assumed they were talking about her. Annabelle wanted to control every little thing Lily did and Stanley would gently convince Annabelle to let go.

Sometimes they would talk about the past. They would talk about Annabelle's early years in this northern Minnesota town. Lily had been able to catch only bits and pieces of their conversations, but it always seemed like there was some unresolved anguish that Annabelle could never truly rise above. She could never be certain, but Lily had always felt like it had something to do with her.

"Would you like some hot tea?" Lily asked Annabelle. Annabelle looked so fragile, so alone. Surely she was chilled to the bone after standing out there on the dock in the biting north wind. But she had said nothing of being cold or sad. Nothing at all about how she felt.

"Yes. That would be very nice." Annabelle seemed to shift to the present. She smiled at Lily. It was a wistful smile that Lily noticed only briefly, not sure of what she saw.

When Lily returned from the kitchen with the hot tea, Annabelle was standing beside the wood stove gazing out the window. Lily paused for a moment wondering if her mother was looking again for Stanley's boat to come in from the lake.

"You are going to miss him desperately, Lily," Annabelle said without turning. "You and I, we have never been close. It's my fault, really. I am so very sorry. I don't know how to fix it." She sounded as though she were on the brink of tears.

Lily was taken aback, too stunned to respond. Annabelle had never said anything like this to her before. Lily continued standing in the doorway balancing the teacup, staring at the back of Annabelle's head. This softness coming from Annabelle made Lily suspicious, and she hated herself for feeling that way.

But then slowly Annabelle turned to look at her, and it was the old Annabelle again. It was the old Annabelle who surveyed Lily critically without saying a word, then took the cup cautiously as though Lily might have put salt instead of sugar in the tea.

"I do believe it's time to check for the red box in the attic, Lily. It could be stored up there. We need to check. I have to find it," Annabelle said, looking past Lily.

"Okay, Mother. I'll get the ladder," Lily answered quietly. She truly wished that they could find this red box so that they could get on with their lives.

"Remorse is memory awake,
Her companies astir —
A presence of departed acts"
— Emily Dickinson

CHAPTER 3

Clancy

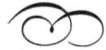

A thin ray of Texas sunlight forced its way through
heavy curtains casting a yellow hue on two elderly
women peering over the top of a tall counter. The women
were as different as night and day. Except for the fact that
they were both exasperated and had reached a level of
agitation where there was no turning back. The larger of
the two women drummed her fingers on the counter's
surface. She glared at the employees on the other side
and made little clicking noises with her tongue, but said
nothing. She wore a faded denim dress, new tennis shoes
with pink socks, and a wide brimmed hat.

The second woman was dressed in a dowdy gray
sweat suit and shiny loafers without socks. Tiny and
skeletal, the second woman wore glasses too big for
her face and could barely see over the countertop. She
placed her hands flat on the on the counter's surface
and started humming. The taller woman twirled the
ends of her hair around her fingertips and began to hum,
too. Their humming was off key and slightly shrill. It
was evident they had no intention of leaving this spot
until their presence was acknowledged. The smell of

cooked cabbage enveloped them. The smell began to flood the room. Finally one of the employees glanced up at them.

"What is it, ladies?" The nurse peered at the two women over the top of her reading glasses. She wore faded green surgical scrubs a size too large, making her appear bony and insubstantial. Pinned to her scrub top was a name tag with the inscription *Clancy Finch R.N.* Her auburn hair tumbled in a loose braid down her back. She was annoyed by the interruption and, without waiting for a reply, resumed making notes on the papers in front of her.

"We need to know when the next bus arrives," the tall woman said simply, almost whispering. She tipped her head slightly forward as if to appear more earnest in her request.

"There is no bus, Doris," Clancy said wearily, barely looking up.

"Oh, well, there must be some mistake. I need to get home. My mother is waiting for me!" Doris's spoke with a sense of urgency in her voice. She brushed stray white hairs away from her eyes and looked searchingly at the nurse.

The tiny woman stepped forward. She smiled politely, admired her fingertips for a moment, then looked around as though she were seeing her surroundings for the first time. Her expression changed into a scowl. "Golly, I never had supper! I am so hungry. I haven't eaten anything since yesterday. Could I just have a little cracker, maybe some milk? Please, anything!" Her tone became more frenzied.

"Muriel, you need to go sit down. Your lunch will be here in a few minutes," Clancy answered, again without looking up. The smell of steamed cabbage was beginning to overwhelm the room. Muriel frowned, covering her nose with her hands.

"Please dear, the bus?" Doris asked again, although this time she was nearly shouting.

"Crackers, milk and crackers, surely you have some!" Muriel screeched, now angry and red faced.

A piercing buzzer startled Clancy. Looking up from her paper work, she yelled to a large Hispanic man dressed in blue scrubs, "Carlos, go check the back door!"

"Huh?" Carlos grunted, distracted by some unseen task.

"The alarm, Carlos! Check the door. Did someone get out?" Clancy's shouts became more exasperated.

Carlos turned and trotted heavily down the hall to the back door, opened it and looked out. Seeing nothing, he punched numbers on a keypad next to the door. The alarm stopped abruptly. He looked back at Clancy and shrugged.

Clancy frowned at him. She looked around, making a mental note of the people in the room. The room was large. It had only one window and a glass door leading out into an overgrown courtyard. Very little daylight found its way into the room. There was a long table with chairs where several elderly people sat quietly. A few of them had their heads on the table and were snoring. There were mauve colored easy chairs occupied by a few other people. Down the hallway leading from the room were more rooms with open doors.

Carlos was slouched against a linen cart in the center of the hallway. He was joined by two nursing assistants dressed in printed scrubs. Clancy was certain one of them had accidentally triggered the alarm. It irritated her. They were talking in Spanish and laughing. Clancy understood just enough Spanish to know that they were discussing whether it was worse to park their cars under trees where the steady onslaught of bird crap would eventually corrode the paint, or park in the blistering

Texas sun where the car's surface would bit by bit turn chalky, then fade to a pastel color.

"Carlos, where's Dr. Finley?" Clancy shouted. She had made note of everyone except Dr. Finley who had a tendency to bolt out any open door when he got a chance.

"*Aqui, aqui!* Nurse Clancy—*Señor* Finley, he is here," one of the women with Carlos shouted. She pointed to the doorway of a room just as a white-haired man with sharp brown eyes shuffled out into the hall. He stood for a moment next to Carlos as though waiting for instructions.

Clancy felt a tug on her arm. "Do you know when the bus arrives?" Doris asked. Her eyes were wide and pleading.

"Doris, there is no bus!" Clancy answered more sharply than she meant to. Softening her voice she said, "Look, your lunch is here. Why don't you and Muriel sit over there and I'll bring you something to eat? Okay? Please?"

"Who is Muriel, dear?" Doris's face clouded. "No, no, I'm not hungry! I can't miss that bus! My mother will be waiting." She spoke firmly, then started to whimper. Her whimpering turned to little breathless sobs.

Clancy didn't answer. Instead she walked from the nurse's desk to the far side of the room and turned on the stereo to the sounds of the Glenn Miller Band. The big band horns and drums pounded through the room. A few of the people sitting at the table looked up, squinting. Smiling at this, Clancy turned up the volume. The music was loud and brassy. Doris stopped crying. She smoothed her skirt and smiled. She was suspended in time.

Doris and Muriel locked arms and strolled over to the stereo. The two of them began to dance. At first they were timid and moved slowly, but as the music blared they began to kick up their heels and swing their hips. They were girls again. The bus could wait. Crackers and milk could wait.

Clancy noticed that Dr. Finley had not left his place beside the linen cart. He stood with his arms at his side and stared into space. Even with the overhead lighting, the hallway seemed dark and shadowy. Ernest Finley looked gray faced and fragile in the dim light. And yet, Clancy could see strength in his dark piercing eyes that made him appear substantial. She could tell he'd been a gentleman. He had been a handsome man. She knew he had been an internal medicine doctor and that he had no family, no friends, no one. No one ever came to see him. His world was this Alzheimer's unit, and he held on fiercely to what he remembered of himself as though he was slipping into mental quicksand.

It was a kind of quicksand, Clancy thought. She looked back at the others as they were served lunch. The smell of cooked cabbage was so pungent now that she wanted to gag. The residents didn't seem to notice. Their sense of smell had dulled with age. Muriel had almost stopped eating completely. She had trouble swallowing because of the little strokes she'd been having over the last three months. She had to eat a special diet of institutional baby food. It was downright disgusting, and yet Clancy had to coax Muriel and the others to eat. They had to eat, didn't they?

Clancy watched as the residents picked at bites of pie or clamped their mouths shut when the nurse aides tried to feed them heaping spoonfuls of meat and potatoes. If they didn't eat, they would become sick from some illness associated with malnutrition, and they could die. Yes, they could die, Clancy thought. Then they would miss their individual journeys through the darkening quicksand that waited for each of them. She shuddered.

"Ernest? Dr. Finley? Come over here and have your lunch." Clancy watched as he did as he was told. He smiled and patted her hand as he passed by her. He rarely spoke.

He sat next to Doris who was staring at her lunch tray. Her chest was covered with a huge white bib. She stared at her plate of food. In her right hand she held her spoon in the air. For a long moment she looked from the spoon to her plate, then back to the spoon. She became more and more frustrated, waving the spoon around. Finally she blurted, "How— am I supposed to eat with this in my hand?"

"That's your spoon, Doris!" Carlos said. He was attempting to shovel food into the mouth of an unwilling bald man wearing giant glasses. The massive glasses were smeared with a thin film of food from previous meals. The other nurse aides rolled their eyes, then resumed talking to each other in Spanish.

Suddenly Muriel began to cough uncontrollably. The cough overtook her. Her whole body trembled, her face coloring from crimson to blue. Everyone gaped at her. By the time Clancy got to her side, the coughing had diminished to tiny hiccups. Muriel looked up at Clancy. "Oh, hello. Can I get you something, dear?" she whispered through the little choking noises.

"What—me? Can you get *me* something? I'm okay, are you?" Clancy laughed.

Clancy might have left this job long ago if it hadn't been for the innocent moments of unexpected humor. Her life away from work had recently become more solitary, more solemn since her parents had died eight months before. They'd died only a month apart. Her mother had struggled with cancer first, and then her father with heart problems. She had moved ahead with things quickly, simply tucking the grief inside to tackle at a future date, not wanting to face the loss.

Lately her free time was spent creating sculptures from soapstone. Her house was cluttered with them. She had no real desire to sell any of it, although some of the pieces were very good. She took classes on stone and marble sculpting and how to turn junkyard finds into beautiful three-dimensional pieces.

Her ten year marriage had been a bitter battle of egos and had failed six months before her parents had passed away. Her husband had told her he'd had enough of her obsession for controlling every little thing. The man had no spine, Clancy concluded the day he walked out for the last time. She watched him leave and felt nothing. Their friends had taken his side, of course. They were exactly like him.

Now at age forty, Clancy had only a few social contacts outside of work. A few women friends from previous jobs. An ex-boyfriend with no demands. The sculpture group she met with once a month. It was enough.

Once she'd been pretty. Really pretty. People complimented her on her looks regularly until she finally found the compliments downright boring. Perhaps in a way she'd just let herself go. Her life wasn't about her looks anymore. She had been a nurse too long, she thought. She'd always cared deeply about her patients to the point of bending rules if she needed to. Still, it was too much sometimes. Sickness and death and suffering. Just too much.

After she'd been fired from her critical care nursing job at the hospital, she took the charge nurse position in this Alzheimer's unit because it was the only position offered to her. She'd been worried she wouldn't find any other work. And maybe, just maybe she needed a less challenging position anyway.

She'd been furious with her supervisor at the hospital. The woman was an idiot anyway. Clancy had yelled—no—screamed at her, telling her that she had no clue how to manage nurses and no clue how to put patients first. She'd told the woman that she was an unskilled, pink-collar piece of protoplasm. And then, Clancy had used brazen profanity that had echoed through the hospital corridors. The other nurses had looked away in embarrassment, but later they thanked her for standing up for them.

Clancy always spoke her mind. She wasn't about to be intimidated by anyone. She had no hesitation in pushing back no matter who it was she might be pushing. Anything less was a waste of time. It had not been the first time she'd been fired from a nursing position for insubordination. Probably it wouldn't be the last.

But the Alzheimer's facility was different. She rarely saw the administrative staff and suspected it was because they were too driven by finances and appearances. She had developed strong attachments to her patients. They seemed to need her loyalty and devotion. They needed an advocate. Just when she thought she'd had enough of their world, they would make her laugh out loud despite the sadness of it all. And no authoritative person had interfered with her work style. Not yet.

Her thoughts were interrupted by a persistent tapping noise. A woman stood at the outside door of the locked unit peering in at her. She looked uneasy and stopped tapping when she caught Clancy's eye. Evidently she doesn't know the code to the outer door Clancy thought, realizing that she had never seen this woman before. She wasn't one of the usual visiting family members, certainly not an employee or a lost administrative person. She looked more like a long-forgotten movie star from the 1940s.

Besides being tall with a posture that made Clancy quickly correct her own slouch, she had frosted blonde hair and was impeccably dressed. She wore a fashionable red suit made of expensive material, and a pearl necklace with matching earrings that appeared to be genuine. Her makeup was flawless. She had high cheekbones and large heavily lashed brown eyes. Her hair was medium length and loosely tied back in a white silk scarf.

The movie star woman had a perfect figure for her age and the most crimson colored fingernails Clancy had ever seen. Her fingers were long and had obviously been manicured for decades. Clancy hid her own stubby clipped nails and antiseptic scrubbed hands. As she studied the woman more closely, Clancy noticed that the woman's hands sagged with wrinkles of a seventy-year-old woman, although she could have easily passed for twenty years younger. She was attractive in a magazine photo sort of way.

Clancy watched as the woman lifted her chin impatiently and tossed her head, patting her lavish hair into place. Actually, thought Clancy, as she went to open the door for her, she looked more like a very wealthy madam. Surely she was in the wrong place.

"Hello. Can I help you?" Clancy opened the door just enough for the woman to decide whether or not she really wanted to enter.

"I'm here to visit Ernest Finley," the woman answered simply, brushing past Clancy into the large room. Everyone stared at her.

"Ernest Finley?" Clancy was amazed. She knew he had no family and as far as she knew this was the first visitor he'd had in the year he'd been here.

"Yes, that's right." The movie star woman had a slight southern drawl. It was an elegant musical kind of sound and commanded a certain type of attention. Obviously she knew this. She looked around the room, turned to Clancy and demanded, "Where is he? Is he here?"

"He's in the courtyard," Carlos answered from across the room. He, too, was gaping at the woman. He quickly looked away when she fixed her gaze on him.

"Well, well. Yes, I do see him now. I'd like to visit with him for a bit, if that's all right?" It wasn't really a question. She strode to the door and let herself out into the overgrown scraggly courtyard. Clancy noticed that she grimaced slightly as she passed the table of residents who were quietly finishing their lunches.

Ernest Finley sat on a rickety wooden bench staring into space as the woman approached. A soft breeze carried her perfume towards him. It was a brilliant late March day, and he had to shield his eyes to see her. He stood up, teetering slightly in his uncertainty.

Clancy watched as the movie star woman embraced Dr. Finley. She couldn't tell if he recognized the woman, but it was clear that he was trying to be courteous. He backed away from her and smiled. She took his hand and together they sat on the bench while the woman spoke to him intently. It was hard to tell if he was actually answering her. He nodded his head and would laugh lightly as he looked up at the sky. Once he uncharacteristically threw back his head and laughed heartily.

Eventually the woman took a white handkerchief from her purse and dabbed at her eyes. She was crying. No, sobbing. She was openly sobbing, and Dr. Finley clearly didn't know what to do. He patted her shoulder and then began to pat her on the head as though she were a child or a hurt puppy. This seemed to make her cry even more, which made Dr. Finley anxious. Clancy started towards the door but stopped herself. She watched as the woman abruptly left his side, walking quickly to the door without looking back. By the time she entered the room, her tears had subsided.

"Everything okay?" Clancy tried to appear nonchalant.

"How is he, really?" The woman drawled in her melodic accent, ignoring Clancy's question. She looked a little drained.

"He really hasn't changed much since he came here. Dr. Finley's such a wonderful man. He seems pretty happy, actually." Clancy was purposefully vague.

"No, I want to know, how is he? I mean, medically? He's so very different. You see, he thought I was his mother." A tiny sob escaped her, but she recovered quickly. She took a pair of dark glasses from her purse but did not put them on.

"Oh, well, yes. You see I really can't discuss that with you. His responsible party is an elder social service agency," Clancy said. Then suddenly curious, she asked "Are you a relative?"

"I don't understand. Surely you can tell me how he is. It's very important that I know. He's—" her voice trailed away.

"No, really, I can't. I'm so sorry. There's a law that prevents me from discussing the patient's condition with anyone but the responsible party." Clancy hoped this sounded kind but could see that the woman was angered by her words. And it was clear she wasn't going to reveal anything about herself or her relationship to Ernest Finley. In fact, she turned away from Clancy to watch Dr. Finley stroll around the weed infested courtyard, stopping every few steps to look at some unseen thing on the ground.

"Ernie..." she murmured, dabbing at her eyes again.

"Clancy! Muriel is on the floor!" Carlos shouted from the hallway.

Clancy groaned. Taking a last look at the movie star woman, she turned and sprinted down the hall to Muriel's room. The patients were always falling. The facility was restraint free, so it was difficult to prevent.

It happened so fast. They lost their footing, someone shoved someone, they became suddenly weak or were attempting to do some unreasonable maneuver.

Once Doris decided to sit on a rolling table. She'd skateboarded along for a minute and seemed to be enjoying herself thoroughly until she collided with the wall and plunged to the ground. Amazingly, she was only slightly bruised. But then, Doris was strong as an ox. Muriel was frail. Really frail.

A small group of residents crowded the door to Muriel's room. Clancy had to gently push them aside, thinking how ghoulish they looked standing there. Doris grabbed her arm. Clancy could see that her face was pale with an expression of silent horror.

Doris adored Muriel. Even though she never remembered her name, they were nearly inseparable.

Clancy looked past Doris and saw Muriel, tiny and crumpled on the cold linoleum floor in a pool of blood. She wasn't moving.

"Clancy! We can't find Dr. Finley!" One of the nursing assistants raced into the room but stopped cold when she saw Muriel on the floor.

"Carlos! Go get one of the nurses from the skilled nursing unit. Now! Somebody, get some towels and ice packs and hurry. Go, go! She's a full code. Somebody else needs to start looking for Dr. Finley. I can't leave Muriel." She shouted orders as she bent over Muriel and checked her pulse and respirations. Okay. She was breathing. The blood was coming from a deep laceration above her right eye. She must have hit her head on the bedside table. A huge lump was beginning to form on her forehead.

"Muriel? Can you hear me?" Clancy wiped Muriel's face with a towel the nursing assistant brought her. She had blood spatters on her scrubs and her hands were bloody.

"Get me up." Muriel answered weakly without opening her eyes.

"Oh crap! What happened?" a nurse entering the room asked.

Clancy didn't recognize the nurse but figured she must be one of the new nurses from another unit. She looked young and inexperienced and did not budge from the doorway.

"Isn't there another nurse working over here?" the new nurse asked, looking back down the hallway.

"Quit. She quit. Actually kind of a long time ago. They just haven't replaced her. I don't think they're trying very hard." Clancy was becoming irritated when she sensed the young nurse's reluctance to help.

"So it's just you working over here? Alone?" she asked, incredulous.

"No choice. Look, I have to call Muriel's doctor. He'll probably want to send her to the hospital. She has a head injury—a bad laceration. She'll need stitches. And I'm sure her hip is fractured." It was a bad fall. Muriel didn't seem to realize the pain yet though. Clancy patted her hand to reassure her.

"Get me up...," Muriel muttered again.

"Hip fracture? How can you tell?" Still without moving from the door, the nurse looked at Muriel with new curiosity.

"See how her leg deviates outward? It's pretty obvious." Clancy wondered why the nurse continued to stand at the door. Did she think she was called over as a spectator? "What I need is for you to stay with her while I call the doctor and the ambulance. You'll need to do neurological checks and vitals signs again. She's full code. Try to keep her still. Can you please do that?"

"Well, yeah, okay. A full code? Why in the world would an Alzheimer's patient be a full code?" the nurse muttered to herself. Finally she moved from the doorway to Muriel. She took exam gloves from her pocket and put them on slowly as Clancy turned to leave the room.

As Clancy hurried towards the nurse's desk, she heard Frank Sinatra belting out *Strangers in the Night* from the little stereo in the corner of the day room. One of the nursing assistants must have given the residents a deck of cards because several of them were sitting at the long table holding cards and sipping on little plastic cups of cranberry juice that looked very much like red wine. What was remarkable was that they seemed to actually be playing a coordinated game of cards while they chitchatted. They were really having fun.

As Clancy neared their table, she realized that they were all playing different games. Not exactly traditional card games. Some weren't playing at all. They were holding cards upside down or flat on the table for everyone to see. A few of them clinked their plastic cups together and laughed robustly. One gentleman squared his shoulders, held his cards very privately to his chest and then suddenly spit on the floor. Another kept telling them it was his turn, his turn, his turn. He said this so many times that everyone ignored him.

A large gray-haired woman dressed in black from her blouse to her shoes, was whispering intently to the woman next to her as though they were partners in the game. She would whisper, glance secretly around the table, then openly point at someone. A few of the residents looked up as Clancy passed by the table. They probably think I'm their waitress, she thought, smiling to herself because it was partially true.

"We found him. He's okay, but we can't get him to come back inside," Carlos said, rushing into the facility from outside. "Some visitor let him out when he said he needed to get something out of his car."

"Dr. Finley? He said he needed to get something from his car? Dr. Finley doesn't hardly ever talk!" Clancy was startled.

"Yeah, I know, I know. But, I mean, he did, Clanc. That's what the visitor said. Now he's sitting in my car like it's his. He got really angry when I tried to get him out. A couple of the other aides are with him now."

"Okay. Just have them stay with him until he calms down. I'll be out there after I get Muriel sent to the hospital."

"You'll need to medicate him. He's too agitated." Carlos concluded, sounding overly confident.

"We'll see." Clancy hated chemical restraint. It was used far too often when all that was needed was a little one on one quiet time. Dr. Finley was probably upset by the movie star woman's visit. He was confused, grasping at his past. He was trying not to sink into the quicksand.

After a series of phone calls and duplicating paper work, Clancy returned to Muriel's room to wait for the ambulance to arrive. The other nurse got up to leave. Muriel lay on the floor with an ice pack to her head and a cover over her tiny broken body. She was oddly quiet.

"How is she?"

"Not as responsive. She looks terrible. Her pulse is weaker...."

The ambulance attendants entered the room with Doris trotting alongside them. Clancy didn't have the heart to send her away. She took her by the arm and led her down the hall as the room began to fill with emergency workers and equipment.

"I believe that's my sister in there." Doris told Clancy, nodding her head as if she were trying to convince herself as well.

"It'll be okay. You'll see." Clancy smiled at her. Doris was so attached to Muriel. They followed each other everywhere. Sometimes she said Muriel was her daughter, sometimes her sister, sometimes a stranger. They had just latched on to each other. It had made their journey into the darkness of Alzheimer's disease less frightening. Clancy sighed.

"I'd like to call my son now," Doris said quietly. It was an unusual moment of clarity for her, and she stood firm in her resolve. "Right now, please."

Clancy knew she had to go see about Dr. Finley but decided to make the call for Doris first. Doris's son was so fiercely protective of her. He adored her. Clancy had never met anyone like him. He was kind and sensitive and yet strong in a quiet self-assured way. He was unusually good looking but didn't seem to realize it himself. Clancy thought it made him that much more attractive.

She'd met him once before, when she was working as a critical care nurse about the same time her parents died. His wife had been one of her patients. It was a sad case, one she wouldn't forget. He had been devastated. His wife had had a complicated head injury from a car accident, and she had been just a little older than Clancy when she died. Too young. He was older than his wife by perhaps ten years. There was an unruly teenage daughter who seldom came to the hospital, even towards the end. The teenage daughter had never been to see her grandmother, Doris, as far as Clancy knew. Never.

As she dialed the phone number, Clancy caught a glimpse of herself in a mirror that had been placed strategically by one of the other nurses on the wall beside the nurse's station. Her reflection was haggard and worn out. She made a mental note to remove the mirror later. There were dark circles under her eyes, and she looked gaunt. Tiny wisps of hair had pulled loose from her long braid making her look windswept. She quickly looked away when Doris's son answered the phone.

"Hello? Mr. Parker? This is Clancy Finch, the charge nurse from Rainy Alzheimer's Care Center. Your mother would like to talk with you. She's had kind of a rough day. Her roommate Muriel has been taken to the hospital. Would you be able to talk with her?" Of course he would, Clancy knew that. He was immediately concerned and wasted no time asking questions. She handed the phone to Doris.

"Hello? I've been waiting for the bus. Is my mother there?" Doris began. She stayed on the phone a very long time. Clancy watched as Doris twirled the phone cord between her fingers and glanced around the room. She felt sure that Doris had likely dreaded old age all her life and now that she was old, she had no real awareness of it.

"Jesus loves me, this I know, for the Bible tells me so, yes, Jesus loves me, yes, Jesus loves me..." sang the group of residents who had been playing cards. They sang the song they remembered from their childhoods perfectly. They sounded like angels. The loudest voice belonged to Carlos. He winked at Clancy from across the room. Clancy smiled.

She felt better when she stepped outside to the parking lot. It was a pleasant early summer day, warm with a light scent of wisteria in the air. She stopped long enough to close her eyes and breathe deeply. When she opened her eyes again she saw him. Dr. Finley sat in the driver's seat of Carlos's car looking grim and determined. Next to him sat one of the nursing assistants reading a magazine.

"Dr. Finley? Everything okay?" Clancy gently opened the car door. Unmoving, he glared at her. "Let's go back inside, okay?"

"No! no, no, no, no, no!" He sputtered, his face reddened with frustration and fury.

Clancy traded places with the nursing assistant who rolled her eyes and shook her head. As she slipped into the car, she could almost feel Dr. Finley's exasperation fill the car. She touched his arm lightly. He jerked away as though he'd been assaulted.

"Ernest, are you upset about your visitor today?" Clancy asked.

He didn't reply. He seemed to become smaller, shrinking into himself. She noticed that he was shaking slightly and did not look well. His agitation was making him sick.

"How about we go for a walk? We could walk around the building. It's such a pretty day," Clancy said. She wanted to ask, who was that strange woman who came to see you? What is it about her that has you so upset? Are you angry because you remember her, or because you don't remember her? Or is it that you want to tell her something, and you can't because you are sinking into oblivion? You're sinking and there's nothing you can do to stop it. Are you thinking if you could just follow her out of here, maybe everything would be okay again?

"No! I can't. No, no, no, no!"

Clancy imagined getting behind the wheel of the car and racing into the sunset with all the windows rolled down. Dr. Finley would be laughing while the wind whipped through his thinning hair. It would be that simple. Nothing else would matter. Just the car barreling down the open road, the setting sun blinding them while the wind swirled around in great gusts lifting them further away.

Suddenly Carlos appeared at the car window. "Hey Clanc, we'll get him." With the help of two other nursing assistants, he managed to pry Dr. Finley out of the car and forcibly walk him back towards the building. Clancy watched Dr. Finley tremble with rage. Still, he held his head high, desperately trying to hold on to his dignity. She knew his agitation had reached a point where he would need an injection to calm him down. To give him some peace, Clancy thought reluctantly.

When she returned to the nurse's desk, she noticed that Doris was chatting and primping and still clung to the phone, which was now upside down. When she took the phone from her, Clancy realized that there was no one on the line. Doris was having a pretend conversation. Well, let her. Just let her, thought Clancy, handing the phone back to Doris. But the spell was broken. Doris walked away. She began to look for Muriel.

"Have you seen my daughter?" she asked. Everyone ignored her.

It was nearly sundown, the time of day when the residents became more confused, more agitated. Clancy had always imagined that they must feel the impending darkness of night descending on them like a cloak. They made her think of flocks of frenzied birds flying in erratic pointless patterns as menacing black clouds of a Texas spring storm rumbled in to devour them. It was that same restlessness. That same helplessness.

She gave her report of the day's events to the oncoming night nurse and began to mentally detach herself from the place. She would go home and shower until there was no more hot water. All the complicated layers of other people's lives would wash into the drain and she could rest. She would remember who she really was while she looked around at her soapstone sculptures and pet her cat. The cat would stare at her knowingly with those big yellow eyes, willing her to unwind. She'd always found that oddly soothing.

"Clancy! Are you listening?" The night nurse's voice jolted Clancy out of her reverie. "The family called while you were outside with Dr. Finley. Muriel died on the way to the hospital. Closed head injury. Nasty business. This is going to be hard on Doris. She's probably going to be difficult. You know how she can get."

Clancy looked over at Doris who stood across the room gazing out the courtyard window at the darkening sky. She was humming *Strangers in the Night*. Her arms were folded tightly across her stomach as she rocked slowly on her heels. She looked horribly lost. Ernest Finley, still a little groggy from his injection, shuffled over and stood beside her. He was already dressed for bedtime in plaid flannel pajamas. He spoke inaudible words, nodding knowingly at Doris. It was as though he somehow knew that she had lost her mother, daughter, sister and best friend all at that very moment. He couldn't have known. Doris waved him away as though he was an annoying insect. But he didn't move. The two of them stood there solemnly as the daylight dimmed.

*"Out of this tangle of threads
to find the thread
that will untangle the threads"*
— Sister Maris Stella

CHAPTER 4

Annabelle

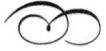

Annabelle gazed intently at her reflection in the mirror. She dabbed dots of cream under her eyes, smoothing it into her skin with small circular motions. The cream was sweet smelling, almost edible. Ignoring an impulse to lick her fingertips, she took a lingering sip of wine from a crystal glass that sat precariously at the edge of her dresser. The wine was warm, stale. She could not remember when she'd poured it into the glass. She took another sip. The bitter taste caused her to gag slightly.

She walked to the window and looked out. She adored this view from the second story window. It had been hers since she was a small child. The large window opened out onto the lake, allowing a misty summer breeze to embrace her. On the beach below, she saw her husband Stanley and their daughter Lily sitting at the edge of the lake It was July sixth and Lily's sixth birthday. Lily was dressed in her favorite plaid shorts and white tee shirt. She had kicked off her sandals and was burying her toes in the sand as she grabbed at locks of her short cropped hair being tossed around by the lively lake breeze. Stanley had delighted Lily by telling her that this birthday was her one and only golden birthday. "You'll only be six on the sixth of July once in your whole life," he told her, winking.

Annabelle watched her husband and daughter throw their heads back and laugh over a shared joke. Stanley had a careless brilliance about him that Annabelle had fallen for years ago. And yet, there was nothing careless about him; he was solid and predictable.

Suddenly Stanley looked up and noticed Annabelle framed by the window. He waved happily. Lily looked, too, but did not wave. Instead, she shaded her eyes and seemed to be yelling a greeting while she pointed to what appeared to be a small fort she'd constructed from beach stones. Annabelle laughed and waved back at them.

She'd made a white frosted angel food cake, decorating it with little paper umbrellas and *Happy 6th Birthday Lily!* written in script across the top. It was perfect. Lily would love it. Annabelle had invited Lily's little friend Tess to the celebration despite the fact that she regarded Tess as a potential problem. The child seemed to have a wild streak that Annabelle did not want Lily to mimic. And yet Lily, too, had her own streak of recklessness. Annabelle had watched this, but had so far been able to control it. There was this daring way Lily approached life that was so unlike Stanley's cautious deliberate manner. The two were so different, and yet they had an unwavering adoration for each other.

In the fall, Lily would begin school and there would be new influences in her life. Stanley repeatedly told Annabelle that she would need to loosen her hold of the child. Let her live life. They would be moving to Texas before then, away from Annabelle's childhood home in northwestern Minnesota. Annabelle was relieved by this. Her own parents had moved long ago to the Black Hills of South Dakota. There was almost no trace left of them. It was as though their dark existence had evaporated from this piece of earth forever. It would be good to move Lily away. She would never have to know about her grandparents.

Annabelle stared again at her reflection in the mirror. Only twenty-three and she already had a six year old child. She shook her head and sighed. She applied red lipstick, then lightly blotted her lips with a tissue. Her long hair was pulled into a French twist as usual. She'd decided the hairstyle made her appear more motherly, more capable. Sort of an Audrey Hepburn look. Looking down at her outfit, she realized that she was still wearing the floral print apron she'd put on that morning over her black pedal pushers and white blouse. Too frumpy for Audrey Hepburn, she decided.

Just as she was considering changing to a summer dress, she heard a knock at the door downstairs. The old clock that had belonged to her grandparents chimed from its place on the staircase wall as Annabelle descended the stairs. She glanced at it. 4:30. Tess was early. The knock persisted.

"Coming," Annabelle called. She flung open the door to Tess and her mother standing on the front porch. Tess held a present wrapped in a multitude of bows and ribbons that clashed with brightly colored paper. Annabelle knew Tess must have wrapped it herself.

"Hi Annabelle, we're a bit early, I'm afraid—" began Tess's mother who stood a few steps behind Tess, her car keys dangling from her hand. "I'm going to have to run. I've got an appointment. Wish Lily a happy birthday for me, will you? Six years old! Can you imagine? The little darling." Without waiting for a reply, she turned and sprinted towards her car. She waved and blew kisses as if this would excuse her hasty departure.

"Hi!" Tess looked up at Annabelle and grinned. The grin seemed slightly impudent to Annabelle, but she found herself smiling back at the child as she welcomed her inside.

"Where is everyone?" Tess peered around corners inquisitively.

"You're the only guest, Tess, just you," Annabelle answered, certain she had already told Tess's mother that Tess was the only one invited.

"Oh," Tess said. It was hard to tell if she was disappointed or relieved.

"Lily is down by the beach with Mr. Storm. We won't be having supper for another hour. Why don't you girls play for a while? Here, I'll take this absolutely gorgeous present," Annabelle said.

Tess beamed as she handed the present to Annabelle, then darted away, the screen door crashing shut behind her. Annabelle saw that the underside of the present had been taped excessively and that some of the bows were a series of knots grouped together. It was actually quite ugly. She placed it on the tea cart next to Lily's other gifts.

It was a glorious day for a birthday. Warm and sunny, with a sky so blue it almost hurt Annabelle's eyes. The table was set. Dinner was already made. Lily had asked for spaghetti marinara, her favorite meal. Simple food for an expert cook like Annabelle. Well, Lily could choose her birthday meal, couldn't she? It was, after all, her day and she was already six years old. School age. Her little girl was already old enough to begin school. As Annabelle continued to marvel at this, she selected a record, a Mozart violin concerto, and placed it on the record player. The melody drifted through the open windows causing Stanley to glance towards the house and smile. Annabelle felt a surge of contentment. She felt protected, safe.

She settled into the plump cushions of the sofa to examine the latest copy of *Life* magazine while she listened to Lily and Tess squealing and laughing on the beach. She turned several pages then looked up at the room around her. She'd decorated the living area and the adjoining dining room with red and white streamers and confetti. The table was set with the red checkered tablecloth that Lily liked so much. Annabelle had even placed tall white candles as a centerpiece, making it all look like their own little festive restaurant. Lily hadn't seen decorations yet. Annabelle smiled, thinking how pleased Lily would be.

The girls came bounding in behind Stanley when Annabelle called them for supper. Tess had evidently already told Lily about the decorations, which made some of her enthusiasm seem contrived. Well, what did it matter? Annabelle seated her daughter at the head of the table. She called her Princess-Lil-the-six-year-old-girl, which sent Tess and Lily into an uncontrolled giggling fit. Stanley gave Lily a little bow and asked her highness where she would have him sit. She pointed to the chair across from her at the far end of the table. She held her chin high and used a serving spoon to point where each of her subjects was to sit.

"Will this be to your liking, Princess Lily?" Annabelle asked in a playful falsetto voice as she presented Lily with a plate mounded with spaghetti sprinkled generously with parmesan cheese.

"Spaghetti? You picked spaghetti for your birthday? Yuck!" Tess blurted. Waving her arms dramatically she added, "you could have had any meal in the whole world! Oh my gosh, Lily!" Quickly she covered her mouth with her hands and ducked her head, trying to avoid Annabelle's disapproving gaze.

"I love spaghetti! Everyone does, Tess. Especially how my mom makes it," Lily said. Then turning back to Annabelle she added, "Tess will be sent to the dungeon for a year of punishment after supper if she does not eat every bite of her food." She sounded as though she were issuing a severe imperial ruling.

"A year? Don't you think that's just a bit harsh, Princess Lily?" Stanley laughed. He was lighting the tall white candles as daylight in the room began to dim with the approach of evening.

After they finished their spaghetti, they sang Happy Birthday as Annabelle served Lily the angel food cake, brightly lit with six candles. Lily shut her eyes tightly and made a wish, looking mildly disappointed when she could not blow out all the candles.

"Presents!" Tess announced.

Annabelle rolled the tea cart next to Lily who immediately grabbed the largest gift from the stack. She began to tear at the wrapping when Annabelle stopped her.

"Lily! For heaven's sake. Slow down. Look to see who the present is from first. And you know we always save the paper," Annabelle said, irritated by Lily's impulsiveness.

"Oh, sorry," Lily said sheepishly, momentarily frozen by the change in Annabelle's tone.

"It's okay," Annabelle instantly regretted stopping her. "Look. It's from your dad and me. Go ahead, open it. Let's see what it is."

Carefully, Lily unwrapped the gift box, placing the paper in a neat stack on the table in front of her. Inside the box was a desk set. There was a blotter, pens, pencils, erasers and a writing tablet. There was a wooden pencil box with Lily's name carved on it that Stanley had made and the largest box of crayons she had ever seen. She examined each item with curiosity but said nothing.

"Open another one!" Tess exclaimed, clearly bored with the gift of school supplies.

Lily opened the next present in the same careful manner. She brushed stray locks of hair away from her face and smiled when she saw a pink nightgown folded into a stuffed toy pajama case. The stuffed toy was a poodle-looking dog. It had soft curly ears and beady button eyes. "Thanks, Mom and Dad. It's really cute."

"Open mine next!" Tess said, nearly shouting.

Lily reached for Tess's gift without hesitation. It was impossible to open carefully because of the numerous ribbons and bows and the endless tape. "Mom, I can't save this paper."

"Here, let me," Annabelle took it from her and while everyone watched, she peeled off each piece of tape and unraveled every ribbon until all that was left was a crinkled colorful blob of paper. She handed it back to Lily.

Lily folded back the paper to reveal two boxes. She looked at Tess, who was sitting on the edge of her chair, her eyes wide with anticipation.

"It's two presents!" Tess said as though no one else could see this.

Lily opened the first box and drew in a breath when she saw an array of perfumes, tiny lipsticks, nail polish, face powder and a beautiful hand mirror decorated with little pearls. Before she exhaled, she opened the second box to find a record. It was an Elvis Presley record, "Heartbreak Hotel." Elvis Presley!

"Tess, I love this—oh my gosh—I'm going to put this stuff on right now!" Her face glowed.

"Oh no. No, you are not," Annabelle said in a quiet, firm voice as she stood up. She took the gifts from Lily and remained suspended as though she was battling an internal conflict almost too huge to bear. Everyone stared at her.

"Thank you, Tess, but Lily cannot accept these gifts. She's far too young for makeup and Elvis." Annabelle placed the lids on each box and handed them to Tess.

"Annabelle—" Stanley began, but stopped when Annabelle glanced at him, her eyes cold with resolve.

"That's not fair! Tess gave me these presents! It's my birthday! It's not fair! Why can't I have them? I'm six years old now." Lily was red faced and angry. She reached across the table and grabbed at the boxes. The perfume box fell open, scattering the little bottles to the floor. Tiny lipsticks rolled to hiding places under the table. The mirror hit the floor with a small thud, knocking some of the little pearls out of place.

"Now, wait a minute, Annabelle, this can't possibly cause Lily any harm. It's just an innocent gift." Stanley jumped up and began to pick the little bottles off the floor.

"No, no it is not. I'm sorry, Tess, I really am. But Lily cannot have things like this. It was very nice of you, but you must try to understand." Annabelle kept her voice low and resolute as she watched Tess's expression change from shock to anger back to shock. There was no way she would ever be able to make the child understand.

Suddenly Lily burst into tears. She put her head on the table, her hair falling into the plate of angel food cake, and sobbed unintelligible words about how unfair it was, how her birthday was ruined. Some of the cake's frosting was smeared into her hair.

"I'm going to take Tess home," Stanley said. He was grim faced and quiet. Annabelle knew that he would find a way to cheer up Tess on the ride home. He was good at that. Good at making people think they understood things they really didn't.

"Bye Tess," Lily whispered through little hiccups. Her face was crimson colored and puffy. She had big globs of cake frosting in her hair. Her eyelashes were wet and matted. She was the picture of misery. Annabelle wanted to go to her and explain to her the things she didn't know. She wanted to tell her that she was still her Princess Lily, that she would always protect her, that it was her job as her mother to mold her into the best person she could be. There were things she would never understand, things she could never know.

She watched as her daughter stood up from her place at the table, her chair scraping the floor as she pulled it back, her small frame rigid as she turned to leave. Annabelle watched in silence as Lily walked away without looking back, her footsteps ascending the stairs as the clock chimed. Footsteps padding into her room. The creak of her bed as she plopped down onto it. Annabelle wanted to go to her. But she knew she would have to tell her more than she wanted to tell her. It would make things worse, wouldn't it?

She heard the car pull away. Stanley would be back soon. She looked at the room again, as if seeing it for the first time. The table was cluttered with spaghetti and cake dishes. There were the festive decorations, the half eaten cake and the tall white candles, still burning. The presents in a heap on the tea cart. The neatly folded wrapping paper. She needed to start cleaning things up, but instead Annabelle covered her face with her apron, unable to cry. She felt as though she was being choked by inertia.

*"I wonder if it hurts to live,
And if they have to try,
And whether, could they choose between,
They would not rather die"*

— *Emily Dickinson*

CHAPTER 5

Clancy

A shrill ringing sound forced its way into Clancy's nonsensical dream. The dream truly made no sense, but it was so whimsical and calming that she struggled to cling to the essence of it. She was powerless to keep it from slipping away as the ringing phone bored into her consciousness. She groaned, pulling the pillow over her head. She waited. After four rings, the answering machine picked up the call.

"Hey Clanc. Where are you? Sleeping? Well, wake up. It's Carlos. Just calling to warn you that the supervisor is going to call you to come in to work. I know it's your day off and you've been filling in a lot lately, but staffing sucks today. We're really short. I'm supposed to be working another double, and there's no nurse scheduled for the afternoon shift. If you don't come in they'll probably bring in some horrible agency nurse. Call me." Click. Gone. A call to warn of another impending call.

Clancy rubbed her eyes and glanced at the clock on the bedside table—6:30 A.M. What was Carlos thinking? He could be such an idiot. There was a time when she thought his attentiveness towards her was a overture to something more amorous until she spotted him one day after work locked in an embrace with his boyfriend. She'd been mildly appalled, but utterly relieved. And yet for some odd reason, he continued to hound her as though he somehow needed her acknowledgment. Maybe it was some unresolved mother issue. Clancy sighed.

She pulled the covers over her head, listening to the steady patter of rainfall on the roof. It was her first day off in two weeks. If the staffing was a disaster, how was that her fault? Maybe if they paid the nurses better or the working conditions were more tolerable, they would be able to keep staff nurses.

Anyway, working with Alzheimer's patients was definitely not for everyone. It was only for those willing to selflessly enter their psychologically complicated world. In a way, people with the disease were like complex children that had been watered down to their simplest form, Clancy thought. When they are hurt, they cry. When they're happy, they laugh. And when they're angry, watch out. And, even though they supposedly had lost their sense of self, each one had their own unique reactions to how they perceived the world around them.

An hour and twenty minutes later, Clancy reluctantly opened her eyes again. She had fallen asleep to the sound of falling rain and to the images of old people shuffling through space. The rain had stopped. Her cat sat within inches of her face staring at her. She scratched him on the head thinking of what she needed to do today. A whirl of chores, errands and other tasks paraded through her mind. She'd already cancelled a lunch date with her ex-boyfriend so that she could have the day to herself to do what she needed or wanted. She desperately needed time to herself.

Suddenly the phone rang again. Clancy yawned, then stretched and turned to face the answering machine, waiting for the inevitable disembodied voice. As predicted, her supervisor shamelessly began begging her to come to work. Clancy rolled to the end of the bed and yanked the cord from the wall.

"See that Bartholomew? That was easy. Easy, easy, just too easy," she laughed to her cat who still watched her closely. His expression seemed disdainful. Clancy abruptly stopped laughing.

She went to the kitchen to make coffee, with Bartholomew pattering along behind her. From what she could see from the parted curtains, the rain had passed and morning promised to unfold into a warm, sunny day. Possibly even hot for May. The soothing warmth of spring gave way to the stifling heat of summer almost overnight in this part of Texas. Still, a good morning for a run.

She slammed down a cup of coffee, fed the cat and changed into her running clothes. As she was tying her shoelaces, she glanced at the dead phone and sighed. Knowing that someone from the sculpture group might call, as they often did on Saturdays, Clancy grudgingly plugged the phone back into the outlet. The phone began ringing instantly.

"Clancy! It's Carlos again. You okay? They're still looking for a nurse for this afternoon and the night shift, too. Call me. They're talking about calling that loud mouth agency nurse that all of us hate. You know—the residents are afraid of her. She makes them all freaky. Where are you?" Carlos pleaded. He hesitated as though waiting for Clancy to cave in and pick up the phone before he disconnected the call.

"Can't do it, Carlos. Not today. I have to have a break," Clancy said to the wall above the answering machine. She tied her hair back into a tight ponytail, suddenly angry that it was assumed she had no life. She turned away and walked out into the morning.

The air was filled with the pungent scent of freshly mowed grass mixed with a light aroma of honeysuckle. She closed her eyes, lifting her face to the sun to savor the mild warmth of the morning. In a matter of hours, this same warmth would heat to a sizzling temperature that would last until sundown.

Clancy stretched, then slowly started jogging alongside the sidewalk past the old 1940 homes with their big front porches and pristine gardens. Her neighbors had evidently shared flower bulbs, and now, yellow and purple irises were blooming in every front yard, next to stands of sage and Mexican heather. Grackles mingled with mockingbirds, greedily stabbing at bits of cat food left on a front porch filled with an overabundance of plants.

A squirrel scampered across Clancy's path into the street, causing a beat-up old Volkswagen to come to a screeching halt, killing the engine. The cursing driver was passed by two cyclists dressed in full cycling gear. The cyclists were talking to each other in exaggerated voices. One of them glanced back at Clancy appreciatively and waved.

She lived so close to the University that after a short distance she began to see more and more college kids milling around. They ignored her. Clancy loved running through the off-campus housing neighborhood because she felt invisible. She stared openly at a student on his front porch, wearing only boxers, standing in front of a large white canvas. He was waving a paint-laden brush at the empty canvas, as though threatening it with artistic violence. There was loud music coming from a second story window that mingled with the street sounds below, causing everything to sound metallic and brassy, drowning out the morning songbirds.

Clancy slowed her pace almost to walking, as she passed a colorful mural extending the length of a windowless brick building. Suddenly she wished she could live her life as a muralist, traveling town to town, climbing to the top of buildings, chasing block-long images. It was the enticement of creating background drama, scenes that were bigger than life, but somehow went unnoticed most of the time, that intrigued her.

She stopped jogging when she reached the campus art supply store, remembering that she'd planned to resume work on the limestone sculpture that sat in the middle of her back yard. It was a sculpture of a buffalo, strong, solid and not even close to completion. She needed a one-half tooth chisel and some newfound inspiration to begin the task. She made a mental note to call some of her sculptor friends later.

When she finally arrived home, Bartholomew greeted her on the front porch by blocking her footsteps, wrapping himself around her ankles in an attempt to warn her of the steadily ringing phone inside. Clancy shook her head. Instead of going into the house, she walked around to the back yard to study her buffalo sculpture, which sat neglected in the center of a small wooden table. She ran her hand over the limestone surface and squinted, trying to sense the direction of its form. It felt substantial, solid, ready to be born. She closed her eyes and inhaled deeply.

Her concentration was suddenly shattered by the sound of a nearby voice raised in anger. She opened her eyes and listened intently, trying to find the source. The primrose jasmine growing around the perimeter of her backyard obstructed her view of any of the neighbor's back yards. The huge mounding vine had prevented her from meeting any of the neighbors around her in the two years she'd lived in her house. Still, she could hear a muffled voice that seemed to be responding to a louder harsh voice coming from the yard behind her. She waited, thinking it would stop.

"We've been over this before, stupid. Do you just not remember? I'm sick of this. We have to do this now. There's no choice—" the angry voice of a man of indeterminate age screeched.

Clancy could not make out the words from the second person, but she could sense frailty in the voice. Maybe even fear. She was startled by what sounded like a table being overturned, then whimpering, then a small dog barking.

"Your problem is that you're just stupid! No, you're a freaking disaster. I have other things I need to be doing today. I can't keep going over and over this with you. We have to do this now or you're not going to like the alternative," continued the angry voice. Then, footsteps stomping away, a door slamming shut, silence. The whimpering increased to small sobs.

Clancy tiptoed to the back of her yard. She carefully parted a small section of the primrose and peered into the back yard of the neighbor directly behind her. Nothing. Taking stealthy steps, she moved over enough to place herself behind the next yard.

She found a natural opening in the primrose where it grew sparse, enabling her to look directly into a back yard overgrown with shrubs, flowers, plants in terracotta pots and hanging baskets. She noticed a small covered patio, which was slightly obscured by trailing ivy and more potted plants. There, in the middle of the patio sat an impossibly frail man hooked to a portable oxygen tank with a small dog sitting quietly on his lap. The man's head was bowed. He was touching his forehead with one of his skeletal hands while petting the little dog with the other. He was wheezing slightly. The little dog watched him with doleful eyes. The man was whispering something to the dog.

All of a sudden the back door of the house opened with a thud as it slammed against the house. Clancy strained to see the entrance. The twist and tangle of primrose vine pinned her back. She struggled furiously with the branches, pushing her way forward enough to see the back of the house. Finally she could see the other man. He was tall and athletic, possibly in his forties, chiseled dark features, thick black hair. He was wearing what appeared to be an expensive suit and tie. Very polished. Very professional. But there was something dark and iniquitous about him. He was evidently so preoccupied that he didn't notice her peering through the vine, gaping at him.

"Oh please, do not start with the self-pity. I'm not missing my meeting for something as ridiculous as this," the younger man said. He stood directly in front of the older man, blocking Clancy's view of him. Suddenly the younger man shot forward, grabbing at the elderly man, nearly toppling his wheelchair back. The little dog began barking and snapping ferociously.

At the same moment, the primrose gave way. Clancy crashed through, tumbling to the ground in a heap. She immediately righted herself and charged forward toward the two men.

"What in the—?" the younger man was alarmed, then immediately composed himself. "Are you alright? Can I help you?" He feigned concern, moving towards her. His menacing demeanor shifted to smooth politeness.

"What's going on here?" Clancy yelled, her voice sharp and accusatory, causing the man to recoil slightly.

"What do you mean?" the man responded amiably, but his eyes were cold.

"I mean," Clancy snapped, "Why are you yelling at him? Why did you shove him? Why is he crying? Why does he look so terrified? I mean, what makes you think you can talk to him like this? What is wrong with you? He's just a little old man! My god, he's on oxygen." She paused, glaring at the younger man.

"Whoa...now wait just a minute. I do not recall inviting you onto my property. What business is this of yours anyway?" His face reddened. "This is my father. He's a very stubborn man and very demented. He's being transported to a nursing home today—without his annoying dog. You have no idea what's going on here. I suggest you leave. Do you understand?"

"No. No, I do not understand. It might not be my business, but I'd be willing to bet that Adult Protective Services would make it theirs!" Clancy realized she was shouting as loud as she had heard him shout when she'd been on the other side of the primrose.

Suddenly the man's cell phone rang. He held up his hand as if telling her to stand by, but turned and walked back into the house, becoming businesslike and disinterested in Clancy as he answered the call.

Clancy looked back at the elderly man. He was shaking slightly, staring straight ahead. The dog still sat on his lap. She pulled up a chair and sat next to him. The little dog eyed her curiously.

"Wife gave me the dog. Before she died. Ten years ago," the old man whispered, still staring ahead. His voice was wheezy, breathless. "Named him Kansas. He's just a mutt. A good dog, though. Always takes care of me." He petted Kansas on the head with his bony hand. His fingertips were blue. The little dog had a scrappy junkyard look about him, and yet he appeared to be as coddled as any fancy breed dog.

"He's cute. Looks like he sure loves you," Clancy said, then added, "I'm Clancy Finch. I live right over there." She pointed toward her house.

"Son thinks I can't take care of myself. Thinks I'm demented. Got emphysema, that's all. Still sharp as a tack." He grinned slightly and finally looked at her. His breath came in short labored puffs.

"So he's sending you to a nursing home? Today? You're going today?" Clancy asked. Her eyes widened.

"Don't want to," he spoke between little gasps for air. "Can't take my dog. Son's gonna have him put down today. Nothing wrong with Kansas. Son said he's taking him to a shelter, but I know he's not." His eyes became teary. The little dog stared at him adoringly.

"Your son seems to be an extremely impatient man. He's not very nice to you, is he?" Clancy said.

The man said nothing. Clancy felt that he'd suffered a long time. How was it, that in the two years she'd lived here, she had never known this gentle old man was in need of help? She could hear his son still talking on his cell phone inside the house. He had a commanding voice, interrupted only by short bursts of phony laughter.

"Son hates animals," the old man said finally.

"I'm so sorry. Is your son taking you to the nursing home?" Clancy asked. She reached across to pet the dog who seemed wary at first, but then began to wag his stubby tail.

"No. He arranged for some sort of transport—" his voice was broken by a spasm of coughing that turned his lips blue.

"My god, you're serious. Your son is very uncaring—" Clancy stopped as she felt anger rise in her.

"Clancy, is that your name? Clancy?" the old man looked at her directly. He looked exhausted, drained of any shred of life.

"Yes, that's right. Clancy Finch," she answered, realizing this man could not be too terribly demented.

"Clancy, would you take my little dog? Would you take Kansas? He's old but he's healthy. He'll take care of you."

"What? Oh gosh, I don't think I can do that. I have a cat," Clancy said hesitantly. She could hear the man's son inside the house, winding up his phone conversation with jovial fake laughter. How was it possible that he could treat his father with such brazen disregard? There was no doubt in Clancy's mind that she would be making a report to Adult Protective Services. Then she would find out where the elderly man was living. She would visit him there. Make sure he was okay. Keep his horrid son away from him.

"Sure, I'll take him. I'll take your dog. He'll be fine with me. You don't worry about this anymore. And when you get settled, I'll bring him to see you," Clancy said suddenly, surprised at her own words.

The old man reached a withered hand towards her and patted her arm. His eyes filled with tears. He flinched slightly when he heard a car door slam somewhere in front of the house. Slowly, tenderly, he picked up his dog and leaned forward for Clancy to take him.

The back door was suddenly flung open. The man's son appeared, looming in the doorway, adjusting his tie, snapping his cell phone shut.

"You're still here? I thought I told you to leave the property," he said, his voice still booming. He took threatening steps forward, stopping only when he saw Clancy stand up with the little dog tucked under her arm.

"And I thought I told you I am reporting you to Adult Protective Services. Why don't you go ahead and call the police? Do it. See what happens." Clancy's anger had risen to boiling. This son was a despicable monster.

"Look lady, I don't know what my father has been telling you, but I have never laid a hand on him. He's senile. He'd say anything. You can hear how he can't even complete a sentence," he snapped, his eyes blazing with anger.

"He can't complete a sentence because he can't breathe! His mind is fine," Clancy shouted.

"You're interfering. The medical transport is here to take him to the nursing home. You need to back off and give me the dog. Now!" he shouted back. It was clear he was used to people jumping when he said jump.

"First of all," Clancy leveled her voice to a sharp hiss, "The dog is now mine. Secondly, your father is not going with some medical transport service to a place he is forced to call home. I will take him myself since you are evidently too busy wheeling and dealing your way through your big business transactions to take him. And third, even if you never laid a hand on him, which I don't believe, emotional cruelty is just as bad. Either way, Adult Protective Services is going to be called. So, you back off."

All of a sudden the son threw his head back and laughed. It was a mocking laugh, laced with malevolence. His cell phone rang. Turning his back on Clancy, he snapped it open and began talking in an assertive, but conversational voice as he walked into the house. He turned back and stood just inside the door.

"I'm sorry, Mr—", Clancy began, turning back to the old man.

"Mr. Eliot," he whispered, looking down at his lap where his little dog had been.

"Mr. Eliot, I'll take you to the nursing home. Do you know which one, or where it is?" Clancy asked, bending to his level while balancing the little dog under her arm.

Mr. Eliot pulled a business card from his shirt pocket and handed it to her. It was a card from the nursing home with the administrator's name on it. He looked up at her expectantly.

"Okay. I think I know where this is," Clancy said, glancing over her shoulder at the son, still standing in the doorway talking on his cell phone. His expression was contorted into a mixture of distant pleasure and present irritation.

"No." Mr. Eliot whispered before a spasm of coughing shook him.

"No? What do you mean?" Clancy asked. She patted him lightly on the back, waiting for the coughing to stop.

"You go. Take Kansas and go. I'll be okay," he said in a voice so low that Clancy wasn't sure of what he'd said.

"No, it's okay. I'll take you. It's not all that far from here. I can stay with you for a while after we get there if you like." Clancy wondered if he did not understand her intent.

"No, please. I want Kansas to think I'm still here. You know, at the house," he paused, sucking in a stream of air, then blowing it out through pursed lips, "Besides, the son— works hard. Important job. Don't want to make him mad. I'm ready to go. You come see me soon. Let me know about Kansas. You should go. Now. Don't want him to take Kansas. Please, go."

"Oh, well, okay. Are you sure?" Clancy could see that he was. "Okay. But I will come see you soon, don't worry, Mr. Eliot. And I'll bring Kansas," *and, I'll be calling Adult Protective Services* she vowed silently to herself and to him.

Just as the back door opened again, Clancy slipped through the primrose with Kansas under her arm. The little dog whined, then wiggled, trying to free himself, but Clancy held tight. She had every intention of keeping her promise to Mr. Eliot. Even the unspoken one.

As she crossed through her back yard to the house, she paused briefly beside the solitary buffalo sculpture. A twist of sadness overwhelmed her for a moment. The limestone seemed suddenly cold and accusing as though it were demanding how long it would have to be kept waiting.

Much to Bartholomew's horror, Clancy set Kansas next to him on the kitchen floor, gave the dog a quick pat, then walked to the phone beside her bed. The message light blinked furiously while she searched through the phone book for Adult Protective Services. She reached for the phone, picking up it up just as it began ringing.

"Hello?" Clancy answered, forgetting that she'd been avoiding the phone all day.

"Oh my god, where have you been? We've been trying to reach you for hours," her supervisor pleaded. "We literally have no one to work the night shift. We have an agency nurse to work the evening shift. I'm trying to make it through the day shift, but there is no one, I mean no one, for nights. Clancy, please, is there any way you could do this?"

"Yeah, okay. I'll do it. I'll be there," Clancy sighed, feeling her resolve slip away. She hung up abruptly, then immediately picked up the phone again to call Adult Protective Services.

Hours later, just shy of midnight, Clancy punched in the code to the Rainy Alzheimer's Center and entered, feeling emotionally drained. She was met with a cacophony of sounds. Fully dressed residents were ambling around the unit, the clamor of their incoherent babbling overpowered only by blaring rock music from the radio and a raucous wrestling match on television. Even more televisions screeched from individual rooms.

The dining room was in complete disarray, with half eaten food trays, spilled beverages and chairs jumbled altogether, blocking any natural pathway. She saw absolutely no staff anywhere. Doris came from behind her, looking red-eyed and fatigued.

"I like you," Doris said, tipping her head to one side. She smiled at Clancy. Her smile was crooked, something Clancy found endearing.

"I like you, too, Doris, but why are you still awake? Aren't you sleepy?" Clancy brushed Doris's bangs off

her face. Doris shrugged, touching her eyelids as if trying to decide.

"Yes. I'm sleepy." Doris said as she looked around
her, then down at her jumper dress. She lifted her dress
slightly and said, "Isn't this pretty? Pretty, don't you
think?"

"Beautiful, Doris. Just beautiful. Where is everybody?"
Clancy said, knowing Doris had no idea. Clancy looked
over Doris's shoulder to the darkened window where
Ernest Finley stood muttering to his reflection in the
glass. The window was too black to see anything outside,
except for the orange glow of cigarette butts. Ernest followed her gaze.

Clancy thought he suddenly seemed self conscious
as he looked down at his hands, then his feet, then back
at her. He smiled. It was his secretive knowing smile. He
would often do this, then nod his head, slowly scrutinize
his surroundings and turn away, whispering his conclu-
sions to himself. Clancy noticed that his sweat shirt was
on backwards.

"Hello Ernest," Clancy smiled at him. To her surprise,
he reached out to shake her hand. She took it and he
shook her hand more vigorously than she would have
imagined. There was a faint odor of urine on him. Ernest
turned, then strolled away.

"Thank God you're here," Carlos said coming up
behind her in a rush. "What a nightmare. Seriously. I'm
doing everything myself. This deadbeat nurse has all
the residents in a frenzy and all the other aides are out
there smoking with her." He was balancing a stack of
washcloths in one hand and a water pitcher in the other.
He had small beads of sweat on his face causing his hair
to hang in wet strands over his forehead, "C'mon, Ernest,
time for bed." Ernest followed Carlos dutifully.

Clancy watched them walk away. Carlos was leading
Ernest who trudged along until he became distracted,

then resistant. He stopped outside the door to his room to read his room number and name out loud. Carlos glanced back at Clancy and shrugged.

Clancy took off her lab jacket and tied it around her waist. She began going room to room switching off the blaring televisions, except for Mrs. Seymour's, since Mrs. Seymour insisted on watching the twenty-four hour seven day a week shopping network channel. It was never off because Mrs. Seymour, who still had moments of clarity, would become restless, agitated and unpredictable if she did not have continuous access to it. She would shriek curses if it was turned off, and at one time Clancy saw her stare at the disconnected television, gasping, pale faced, unmoving, incredulous that the monotonous parade of lively salespeople had been extinguished. Even when she was sleeping she seemed to need these salespeople telling her what she needed to buy, what items she couldn't live without, over and over again. If it was turned off while she slept, her voice would awaken from under the covers, immediately demanding that it be reinstated. She would say this without moving, without even opening her eyes.

Clancy turned off radios, dimmed hall lights and straightened chairs. She rolled a cart to the tables and began removing trays and dishes. Medicine cups sat beside trays untouched. People were continuing to pace, but more slowly now, as though they sensed the restoration of order. Order and security.

One of the residents began intently wiping the tables with a small piece of tissue. She was humming an unidentifiable gospel tune. Her eyes were closed as she moved from table to table with the tissue in her hand. The woman was morbidly obese and rocked gently on her heels, shifting her weight onto her walker as she stopped at each table. Clancy noticed that the bandage on her arm needed changing. Just as Clancy went to her for a closer look, the woman began to belt out a booming version of *How Great Thou Art,* her eyes twinkling as she watched Clancy approach.

At the same moment, the courtyard door creaked open. The evening nurse and three nursing assistants filed into the room. A waft of rank smoke drifted in with them. They were talking in loud voices, only stopping when they noticed Clancy.

"Oh, hey Clancy. It's Clancy, right?" The evening nurse looked around the room. The chaos she'd initiated during her shift had dwindled to a low hum of activity. "Wow, look at this. Everything quiet. You must be a magician." Her laughter sounded hollow, almost taunting.

"I just need to get report and count narcotics with you, then you can go," Clancy said through clenched teeth. The nurse was a brazen slob. She obviously did not care about the patients. It was just a pay-and-go baby-sitting job to her.

After the evening nurse had given Clancy a scant, unimpressive report filled with omissions, she flounced out the door without a word. Clancy sighed. She made some notes, then stood up to make rounds.

The residents were quiet now. A few had gone to bed and others wandered in the hallway. They seemed suspended in space and time. Clancy wondered how many of them had been brought here by a frustrated family member. Or how many were like Mr. Eliot, leaving behind a favorite little dog and a cruel son who just wanted him out of the way.

How many of them had been snatched out of lives that seemed meaningless to the people around them? How many of them had been cognitive enough to understand that they would never return?

"After unbearable days
Of careful breathing
Heaven waited
In the white light
Of believing
The eyes of joy
Would soon shut tight
Around soft wing beats
Of silence in flight"
— L. Storm

CHAPTER 6

Lily

Hours grew into whole days, expanding into weeks, until nearly a month had passed while Lily continued to help Annabelle search for the red box. They hadn't looked for it every day. They looked for it only when Annabelle became suddenly obsessed with locating it. Lily despised those days. She'd started to believe that there was no red box, that her mother had fabricated it to cause even more friction between them.

But then, there were days when it seemed that Annabelle had simply forgotten about the search for the box. She would become despondent, pacing silently at night, or she would become animated, almost personable, enjoying their strolls in the woods, their shopping trips in town. She seemed to delight in lingering by the boathouse along the water's edge, lake water splashing on her face as she stooped to examine tiny seashells. On those occasions when Annabelle seemed almost childlike, Lily tried to understand this woman who had been her mother.

Lily tried to imagine Annabelle as a child but even as she laughed lightheartedly, sadness was etched into the lines of her face. Worry lived behind her eyes. Something haunted Annabelle. Something hidden in the deepest corners of her soul. Something she had never talked about with anyone but Stanley. It was something that caused her to be suddenly cruel at times and other times disconnected. Once or twice, through swallowed tears, Annabelle would mutter an apology to Lily for something nonspecific. Lily found this so disturbing that she would back away from Annabelle, her emotions frozen.

"Lily? Did you hear me?" Tess's voice interrupted Lily's thoughts. "You really should try this walleye pike. Will's recipe is unbelievable. Lily?"

Lily and Tess had taken Annabelle to the Gray Dawn for supper. Tess's husband Sam and her son Teddy had come along at the last minute. Since Lily and Annabelle were to leave for Texas the next day, they had decided to make it into a special occasion. Annabelle had over-dressed in her Sunday best but didn't seem to notice that everyone around her wore jeans, T-shirts and lightweight sweaters. They'd chosen to sit outside at a table on the deck overlooking the lake.

The early summer air was crisp, even chilly, but so exhilarating that no one mentioned being too cold. Long shadows poured across the front lawn. The sky had darkened to a deep indigo. They watched as the setting sun saturated everything in its path with a golden hue, splashing the sky with pink and orange. The day's parting colors matched Annabelle's dress.

"Okay then, I'll have the walleye," Lily said as she looked up to see Will grinning at her as he made little notes on his order pad. She smiled back at him. His casual manner made her feel totally at ease for the first time in weeks.

After Will disappeared into the café with their orders, Lily glanced around the table, her eyes resting on Annabelle who seemed immensely happy at that moment. She wore an uncharacteristic, extravagant amount of makeup and her long graying hair was an unrestrained mess. Her dress was a batik print, the colors flattering her skin tone. She had been beautiful once with her angular features and long dark lashes over deep-set eyes. There was a sort of Bohemian look about her. Almost like a perennial art student. She had ordered wine and was now taking tiny sips without pausing.

"So," Sam began, "kind of good to be up this early in the season, eh? Before all the tourists, I mean."

"Wonderful," Annabelle murmured without looking in his direction. She swallowed more wine in gulps.

"It had to be terrific growing up in this lake town, Annabelle. You must have a lot of good memories. Nothing bad ever happens here. Really good people live here, salt of the earth," Sam said, tapping his wine glass for punctuation.

"Salt of the earth," Annabelle repeated each word, her tone slightly mocking, then added with deliberate hesitation, "I suppose." She turned away and watched a small cloud drift across the darkening sky.

"So, do you think the town has changed much over the years?" Sam persisted.

"Yes. Well, no. Maybe some things for the better. It wasn't always all good," Annabelle answered. She put her hand to her mouth and looked away. It was clear she did not want to continue.

"Actually, if spring wasn't such a busy time in the gardening business, I'd come up this time of year from now on," Lily said.

"You've been gone from Texas a long time. Probably you'll be really swamped with work when you get back, don't you think?" Tess said.

"Oh yeah, well. The assistant manager has things under control. I talk to him every other day. He's a gardening wizard. It'll be fine. It's good we came up, you know." Lily glanced at Annabelle. She thought of her dad for a moment, how Stanley would have enjoyed being up here for so long. He wasn't overly fond of Texas. But had the trip helped Annabelle with her grief? Lily wasn't sure.

"Gardening business? What do you mean? Gardening?" Annabelle flashed her dark eyes at Lily. Her expression was full of accusation as though Lily had slipped a secret past her.

"Well, yeah. I mean you know that, Mother. I've owned and managed the Green Thumb Garden Shoppe on West Dobbs Street for quite a while now," Lily said, adding, "you've been there once, maybe twice."

"No, I haven't. And you never told me this. I would remember something like that. For heaven's sake, Lily, you're a journalism major. What kind of work is digging in the ground? You're smart, Lily, you need to find something better than that," Annabelle snapped, clearly annoyed.

Lily groaned. Could grief have taken such a toll on Annabelle that she would forget the most basic things? They'd had this same conversation two years ago. Annabelle's grief seemed unnatural. But then, Lily's own grief over the loss of her father was a vast space yet to be filled. She chose not to answer Annabelle. She felt a confrontation brewing. Maybe Annabelle had had too much wine. Lily noticed Tess and Sam exchange quick glances while Teddy stared at his silverware.

Annabelle made a small grunting sound, then drained her glass of wine. She looked embarrassed but recovered quickly when there was a sudden splash in the lake as a small flock of Canadian geese came in for a landing. Everyone looked in the direction of the geese.

No one spoke for a few moments. The silence made the air seem colder, like a patch of ice waiting to be crossed. The geese began to make loud honking sounds, shattering the stillness. Only a faint trace of the sun still dotted the horizon. Pinks and oranges gave way to lavenders and deep blues, colors bleeding together like a watercolor painting. The candle on their table flickered as though waving farewell to the departing sun.

"Did you ever find that red box?" Tess asked, realizing immediately that this, too, was the wrong topic. "Oh look. Look at the first stars. Isn't that spectacular?" she added abruptly, hoping to shift the conversation to something neutral.

"Red box? No, gosh, no. We sure did look. It's definitely not here." Lily laughed slightly, thinking of the ridiculous amount of time and travel spent looking for the box.

"Well, it's somewhere," Annabelle said, her voice low, almost a hiss.

"Probably in Texas, Mother. We'll find it," Lily said irritably.

"So, what's in the box anyway?" Teddy asked looking from Annabelle to Lily, unaware that even Lily had no idea. Everyone looked at Annabelle.

"Oh, various items, you know, letters, documents, insurance policies, old photos, old passports and a diary. Just things important to me and Stanley." Annabelle looked around the table at her audience. Just as she began to dismiss the subject with a wave of her hand, her face darkened. Something in her manner became rigid.

At that moment, Will appeared long enough to serve their dinners, pour more wine, then bid them *bon appetite*. If he had wondered at their silence, he gave no indication.

"Mother? Are you alright?" Lily cut a tiny piece of the walleye pike and put it in her mouth, savoring the flavor. She would not let Annabelle ruin this dinner.

"She stole it, you know. Lily stole the red box. That's what happened. It was a criminal act. And the box is mine, my property," Annabelle's voice was controlled, but daring. She took no notice of the dinner in front of her.

"What?" Lily dropped her fork. It made a loud clanking sound as it hit the plate, scattering bits of rice onto the tablecloth.

"Oh yes, yes you did. That's why we can't find it," Annabelle raised her voice loud enough that a few of the customers dining inside the Gray Dawn looked in their direction.

"So, you're saying that I drove you fifteen hundred miles from Texas to the lake cottage, to find this all-important red box that I'd already stolen? Are you listening to yourself? That's totally nuts!" Lily wanted to laugh.

"I know you took it. I think it's rotten of you to not give it back. You don't understand how important it is to me and to Stanley," Annabelle lowered her voice. She looked as though she might cry.

"Mother, I don't have it. I don't even know what's in it. I don't know what it looks like. I have no idea where you might have put it. Or even if it's actually red, or burgundy or dark pink. Is it luggage, a handbag, a storage chest? I mean what is it, really?" Lily glanced at Tess who widened her eyes and shrugged, but then looked away.

"Don't play stupid with me, Lily," Annabelle suddenly yelling, rose to her feet and pointed an accusing finger at her daughter. She slammed her other hand, open palmed onto the table causing the silverware to jump, as if startled. More customers in the café looked in their direction.

Tess and Sam shifted uneasily. Teddy stopped chewing a mouthful of food, his jaw dropping open in astonishment. Lily sank into her chair, covering her face with her hands.

"I can't do this," Lily said directly to Tess, "I cannot do this." Then turning back to Annabelle she said slowly, quietly, "Mother, I understand that you miss Dad, okay? But Dad's death happened to me, too. I mean, I'm trying to deal with my own grief. This drama of yours is not helping either of us."

"Your father is going to be very angry," Annabelle's yelling advanced into a kind of horrible screeching sound. From inside, people openly stared at her with raised eyebrows, shaking their heads in ignorant disapproval.

Suddenly Lily stood up, turned from the table, her napkin dropping from her lap to the ground and walked back into the café without a word, leaving Annabelle sputtering in the background. Lily took long strides past a table of onlookers, her chin held high, eyes averted.

Thankfully the women's rest room was vacant. Lily entered the furthest stall and sank onto the edge of the toilet seat. Her sobs began to escape into the hollow air as she allowed herself to think her darkest thought. Why couldn't Annabelle have been the one to go first? Why did it have to be Stanley? Why not Annabelle? She let herself imagine this. Actually imagined Annabelle gone. Imagined having her father to herself without his constant devotion and attention to her mother. It would have been so different. So much better. Life would have gone on as it should.

Lily felt a rush of guilt overcome her. She wiped her eyes with the backs of her hands and stared straight ahead at the graffiti carved into the door of the stall. In juvenile script, someone had written, WHERE THERE'S DOPE, THERE'S HOPE, which Lily found odd, wondering what teenage girl might have taken the time to carve this into the paint and why.

The rest room door opened. Someone entered, tentatively. Lily looked under the stall to see Tess's sneakers stopped at the entrance, closing the door behind her.

"Lily? You okay?" Tess asked.

"Yeah," Lily stood up, opened the stall and faced Tess. She rolled her eyes and shrugged.

"Annabelle's fine now. Teddy got her talking about painting. He's showing her his paintings in the café. She seems all happy again. But she doesn't remember Teddy from a few weeks ago. It's like she's just meeting him for the first time," Tess said.

"Oh."

"Sorry I mentioned that stupid red box," Tess said. She glanced at herself in the mirror, brushing unruly blonde curls from her forehead.

"How could you have known?" Lily said. She leaned against the wall, folding her arms across her chest and looked down.

"Annabelle isn't right, Lily."

"What do you mean?" Lily asked cautiously. She looked up at Tess.

"Well, I mean certain things. Her outbursts. Her forgetfulness. I mean it seems disproportionate, you know?" Tess closed the gap between them and was now standing directly in front of Lily.

"No, no. It's my fault. I've not been much help to her, really. Dad would want me to step in and take care of her. You know how he doted on her. She's so incapable on her own. She misses Dad more than breathing. It's so sad. I don't know how to make it better for her and I end up causing problems with the things I say. It drives her to be erratic. She's just overcome with grief," Lily said.

"Or maybe, she had too much wine. You think? She drank that first glass pretty fast for a fifty-two-year-old woman," Tess said.

"That's true." Lily believed this a little. It could have been the wine.

"Sam bought her some coffee," Tess said. "I think it's safe to return. She seems good, you know, fine. We should go finish our meal. We won't see each other again for another year. C'mon."

When they returned to the table, Lily noticed how dark the sky had become. The centerpiece candle continued to flicker and dance, illuminating Annabelle, Teddy and Sam's faces with a soft orange glow. Annabelle was laughing at something Teddy had said. She was wrapped in Sam's sweater against the descending night chill, her hands cupping a steaming mug of coffee. At that moment, Lily thought her mother looked painfully vulnerable, like a woman who had either known the world too well or had not known it at all.

"Lily, this young man Teddy did all the paintings in this café. He's an artist. Isn't that wonderful?" Annabelle said. Her earlier flash of anger had been extinguished. Her smile seemed genuine. She beamed at Teddy as though he were her own offspring.

"I know, Mother, I told you about his paintings last—" Lily stopped herself. Annabelle truly did not remember being told this. She didn't even remember her previous encounters with Teddy. She had just been so preoccupied with the loss of Stanley. Lily could see that now. "Yes, it is impressive, Mother. Really impressive."

Lily vowed silently to be kinder to her mother. More tolerant. More like Stanley would have been. She would help her through this time of grief and somehow in the process they might become closer. Maybe Annabelle would open up to her. Reveal the core of her sadness, explain her severity, her complexities. Lily knew nothing of Annabelle's youth because Annabelle always avoided the topic. For that matter, Annabelle rarely spoke of her own parents. The only grandparents Lily had ever known were Stanley's parents. And they had been such lively, affectionate people that the absence of Annabelle's parents had seemed unimportant.

Before dawn the next day, Lily stood by the kitchen window sipping coffee from the thermos that was intended for their car trip. She parted the curtains. Except for the moon, the sky was black. There was no sign of the day to come. The moon's reflection on the lake was being sliced into turbulent strands of light by the splash of waves. It was soothing, in a chaotic sort of way. Lily jumped slightly when Annabelle came up behind her. She hastily placed the cap back on the thermos.

"You're up early," Annabelle said, rubbing sleep from her eyes. She yawned. Caesar, her old basset hound, padded into the room looking droopy eyed. He plopped down beside Annabelle.

"Well, of course. I mean, didn't we decide we needed to get an early start back to Texas?" Lily said.

"Texas? What?" Annabelle squinted at Lily.

"It's today, Mother. We're going home today. I have to get back to work, remember?" Lily decided Annabelle must still be half asleep and offered her a cup of coffee.

"Oh. We're going home today?" Annabelle repeated. She seemed more baffled than sleepy. She took the cup of coffee but didn't drink. She looked from the cup in her hand to Caesar by her feet, then back to Lily. "To Texas, we're going to Texas?"

"We ought to be able to make it to Kansas City easily today," Lily said, visualizing the map she'd studied the night before, not noticing Annabelle's bewilderment.

"We're going home today?" Annabelle's tone became more urgent. She reached for the tea kettle, went to the sink, filled it with water and returned it to the stove, turning the dial for the burner.

"What are you doing? I already made coffee. We're leaving within the hour, Mother," Lily said, noticing, too, that Annabelle had turned on the wrong burner. Lily quickly switched it off.

"Oh," Annabelle said. She seemed lost, wrapped in Stanley's old terry cloth bathrobe, her hair in disarray, her slippers on the wrong feet. She stared at the untouched cup of coffee Lily had given her that was now sitting on the counter.

"Mother, your slippers..." Lily started but stopped, then began again. "I'm going to finish packing the car. You take your time getting ready, okay?"

The coolness of the early summer morning caused Lily to shiver a little as she stepped outside. They had a long trip ahead of them, and she was anxious to get on the road. It had been good for Annabelle to make the yearly trip back to her childhood home so soon after Stanley's death. The cottage had been their sanctuary over the years. Lily had no doubt that there were memories of Annabelle's youth lurking around every corner, but Annabelle never mentioned anything.

Once though, when they had been grocery shopping in town, Annabelle had reacted strangely to a man who spoke to her as though he'd recognized her from her younger days. When he'd first appeared, Lily and Annabelle had been lingering in the produce aisle picking through the bin of baking potatoes. The selection of potatoes was small, just like the store. The old grocery store had barely changed since Annabelle was a toddler. To Lily it seemed frozen in time, with its creaky hardwood floors, gray with age and footsteps. Neatly placed rows of canned goods, rice and flour led the way to a small bakery and butcher display attended by the jovial proprietors who would always greet and tell customers the specials in the same breath.

When the stranger first spoke to Annabelle, blanched panic shot across her face. She had immediately positioned herself in front of Lily, blocking her from the man. Her demeanor became defensive, protective.

Lily had never seen the man before. She figured him to be older than Annabelle by six, maybe seven years. Even in his late fifties, the man still had an attractive blue collar recklessness about him. He looked as though he'd lived hard, that he'd flirted with disaster more than once. A smoker, likely a heavy drinker, probably even a womanizer, Lily guessed. The man seemed uneducated, but bold and unapologetic, almost defiant. His eyes were weary, but piercing all the same. He was dressed in jeans and a worn work shirt with the local hardware store's logo. Lily remembered thinking that he couldn't possibly have been a friend to her intellectual father. Or for that matter Annabelle, who was so proper and refined.

The man had stopped cold in his tracks, openly staring at Annabelle. Lily had to admit that her mother did look lovely that day with her long graying hair tied neatly back away from her face. Her skin was smooth, but slightly ruddy from so much time spent outside. She was wearing something sporty, which had made her appear energetic, youthful.

"Annabelle? Annabelle Doyle? Is that really you? No way. By god, it is! Man, what a surprise this is. How many years could it be," the reckless man had said, stepping into their space. He was large and loomed over them. Lily noticed that the only items in his grocery cart were a loaf of bakery bread and a six pack of beer.

"It's Storm. Annabelle Storm," was her mother's icy, guarded reply.

"Oh, oh yeah, yeah, that's right, Storm." He had then turned to look at Lily appreciatively. It made Lily uneasy only because of Annabelle's manner, "and this, this must be your daughter? Is that even possible?"

"Yes, this is my daughter. Stanley's and my daughter," Annabelle answered. Her words were precise and sharp. She seemed tiny next to the reckless man, but fierce as she stood her ground, making confrontational eye contact with him.

"Well, isn't that something? She looks just like you, Annabelle. Hard to believe—." He drifted into a memory for a moment, not sure how to get past Annabelle's remote formality. He stroked his chin thoughtfully.

"Uh-huh, well, it's been a pleasure to see you again Frankie, but we really must be going. Good-bye," Annabelle said. Taking advantage of his hesitation, she'd turned quickly, dropping potatoes back into the bin. She took Lily by the arm all in one swift motion out of the store. The two women walked quickly away without a glance back.

When Lily asked later who the man was, Annabelle told her that she really wasn't sure. Maybe Frankie wasn't even his name, she'd said, then changed the subject. Lily couldn't imagine an adult man with the name Frankie. Frankie? Maybe Annabelle was mistaken.

An owl hooted in the tree above Lily. The early morning was so dark, it may as well have been night. She opened the trunk to the car, dropping her suitcases towards the back to make room for Annabelle's things. Annabelle had always traveled with more than she could ever need. Thinking of this, Lily smiled but her smile faded quickly when she picked up Annabelle's suitcase. The weightlessness of it caused her to tip back. She picked up the second bag and the third and found them to be the same. When she looked inside the bags, she was shocked to find them empty. Completely empty. Annabelle had packed nothing.

For a fleeting moment, Lily remembered what Tess had said about her mother. That Annabelle wasn't right, her confusion was disproportionate. But then Lily vaguely remembered that over the last year or possibly years, Stanley had helped Annabelle do most everything, including packing. It was automatic. He seemed to thrive on it. Lily had admired his absolute devotion to Annabelle, never once imagining that Stanley helped her mother because she was unable to do things for herself.

Lily sighed heavily. Stanley wasn't coming back. This was all going to take time. She picked up Annabelle's empty suitcases and walked back into the cottage.

"Still the earth
Would hold me
Without a friend
My only comfort
This world
Of Pretend"
     — *L. Storm*

CHAPTER 7

Annabelle

The early days of June brought rain almost daily. The Texas sky remained colorless, the air oppressive. In the evenings, storms would brew, stirring great violet clouds up from the horizon into towering drifts of ominous vapors. The distant crash of thunder and sheets of heat lightening occurred nearly every night.

It had been two months since Stanley's passing and a week since Annabelle and Lily had returned from the Minnesota lake cottage. Annabelle missed Stanley more than she'd thought possible. She'd never felt so alone, so unsure of herself. When the rains came, it was as though the heavens wept with her.

Most days she was content to sit quietly in Stanley's study and think. Or read. Read books or the newspaper. Her fascination with the paper had more to do with the photos than any of the written text, and the books she selected were usually large colorful travel books. Sometimes she even read some of the poetry Lily had written over the more recent years. The poems were all untitled. If Annabelle had ever understood the poems, she no longer did. But she enjoyed the images Lily could paint with words. And that was all it was for Annabelle, really. Just words. Imaginative words on paper. Her daughter was quite gifted. Had she ever told her this? She could only remember pushing Lily to do her best. Never letting up. Never. It was harsh sometimes, but necessary.

Annabelle's own writing had always been limited to journals. Nothing literary or creative, just recorded observations. Whole years would go by without a single entry, but then there would be an event or a feeling that would draw her out again, and she would write with fervor. Most of her entries resembled a child's diary. Chaotic and full of emotion. She'd intended to destroy them, but never had.

She glanced out the window of the study. The window was ajar. The curtains fluttered with the breeze. It was already nightfall. The rain-scented air mingled with the smell of the old wooden desk and worn books. It soothed her. She noticed an open diary on the desk in front of her as if seeing it for the first time. Putting her glasses on, she read the words she had written earlier in the day.

"All I know is that I know enough to know that I don't know very much," she read aloud, her voice nearly a whisper. She swallowed hard, not knowing why she had written these words. There was nothing else written on the page. She closed the book.

Suddenly Annabelle realized she was famished. She couldn't remember when she'd last eaten. As she pondered this, she became aware of her basset hound shuffling into the room. He whined softly at her feet. Putting his head in her lap, he gazed dolefully into her eyes. She smiled, patting him absentmindedly.

"I bet you're hungry, too, hmmm?" she said, trying to remember his name. At that moment, his name was swallowed up by the darkness of the empty evening. The more she pet him, the more she could not recall her dog's name. She pet him harder and harder until he finally backed away from her.

"How about we go into the kitchen and see if I can find you something to eat, old doggie." She finally decided to call him old doggie. It disturbed her to watch him pull away from her. If only she could remember his name.

The dog followed her dutifully into the kitchen and watched as she opened the refrigerator. He watched as she stood staring at an array of leftover food, meals prepared by someone for her to eat, finally selecting a plate of rice and chicken. She went to the pantry and stood staring even longer. When the dog whined again, she selected a can of pears and began looking for a way to open it.

"Where is your dog food? Don't you have dog food?" she asked Caesar, as if expecting the dog to show her. When he cocked his head to one side and yapped, it startled her.

With more urgency, she looked for a way to open the can. Finally she found a hammer and nails under the kitchen sink. After uncertain deliberation, she began to hammer a large nail into the can of pears. She did this along the entire lid until she was able to pry it off. The jagged lid sliced a path along the side of Annabelle's thumb. Blood gushed from the wound, causing her to pause long enough to wrap a piece of paper towel around her hand. She poured the pears onto the dish of rice and chicken and set it on the floor, giving Caesar a little scratch behind his ears.

"There you go, old doggie."

While the dog ate ravenously, Annabelle began methodically setting the dinner table, her hand bleeding and still wrapped in the paper towel. She took linen napkins from the hutch, the good silver, the Waterford crystal and the best china. Slowly, she began to set ten places, carefully placing each silver piece, each salad plate, each dinner plate. Satisfied that everything was in its rightful place, she walked away, leaving the bloody paper towel crumpled on the table.

The house was dark. Too dark, Annabelle thought. She felt uneasy, almost fearful of the darkness. The darkness and the silence. The only sound she heard was Caesar's tongue slapping across his dinner plate. She listened to this until the predominant sound shifted to small pinpricks of rain on the windows.

"Lily? Lily!" Annabelle's voice echoed through the house. Of course, Lily wasn't there. Annabelle remembered suddenly, but she was coming over soon, wasn't she? She would be there. Lily would be slightly aloof, slightly detached, but she would still be there. She would come. Annabelle began walking from room to room, switching on overhead lights.

She stood quietly beside her bed. It was torn apart, covers swirled together as if in the throes of a nightmare. She found this unsettling, almost frightening. Who had done this? Instinctively she crouched to the floor and looked under the bed. And there it was. The red box. She tugged at it, moving it to her bit by bit. It was smaller than she'd remembered. Too small. But it was the red box. A shoe box wrapped in bright red paper.

It didn't seem quite right. She ripped it open anyway, knowing it contained important parts of her life. Parts of her she had to have back, to hold onto for a moment, savor, embrace, reject, discard. But even as she tore off the lid, she knew it was all wrong. The box was only a present she'd hidden from Stanley last winter. She stared at the contents. New heavy leather gloves sat uselessly at the bottom of the box, the fingers touching in an empty prayer. Stanley had never worn the gloves. She had forgotten to give him the gift. Now, he never would wear the gloves. Annabelle began to cry.

She sat on the floor and sobbed for her dead husband, for herself, for her daughter, for all the sad things of the world. Her heart tried to break. Tried desperately to shatter into pieces. Caesar trotted in to sit beside her. He licked her face. His breath reeked of something like canned pears but Annabelle could not quite place the smell.

The red numbers on the bedside table's digital clock caught her attention as the minute clicked into the next minute. The time was wrong. She would have to fix it. The clock had lost hours and hours of time. She grabbed hold of the bedside table, pulling herself to her feet, still staring at the clock, knowing the time had to be wrong without having any real sense of what the numbers meant. She looked away.

Next to the clock was a large address book tucked partially under the phone. Annabelle picked it up and began to thumb through the pages. The first section included emergency phone numbers, taxicab numbers and still other numbers that meant nothing to her. She turned to the 'S' section and recognized a series of addresses and numbers under the last name Storm. When she came to the name Myrtle Storm, she paused, frowned, then read the name aloud.

Myrtle Storm. Stanley's Aunt Myrtle. It had been so long since Annabelle had seen her. How long? How long had it been? And wasn't Aunt Myrtle the one who had always been so very kind? Had she not always welcomed Annabelle into her home with generosity and warmth?

Yes, of course. And, too, Aunt Myrtle was such an eccentric. She had that huge aviary of doves and finches off of the living room built right onto the front porch. And she had other birds inside the house. They were large talking birds that she'd doted on like babies. Childless, eccentric, spinster Aunt Myrtle. She dearly loved Lily and never forgot her birthdays. The last time Annabelle had seen her, Aunt Myrtle told her to come by anytime. No need to call, she'd said, just come by anytime day or night. So, why hadn't she done that, Annabelle wondered. Why had it been so long?

She studied the address. It was unfamiliar. But it was in Georgetown, just north of Austin. Not that far, really. Annabelle knew she would lose her direction. She hated driving to unfamiliar places. But she should go. It would be so good to see Aunt Myrtle again. Of course Aunt Myrtle must surely know about Stanley by now. She would want to know. He was her great nephew, after all.

She decided to call a cab. She jabbed in the phone number for Blue Cab Company and listened. When the dispatcher answered, Annabelle said she needed a cab right away. Then slowly she read Aunt Myrtle's address into the phone.

"Okay. Okay, yes ma'am, but where do you need the cab sent to? I mean, where you are now?" the dispatcher said impatiently.

"Oh. Um, well, wait a minute. It's here somewhere." Annabelle fumbled with the address book, suddenly nervous. She read the address she found on the inside cover to the dispatcher. "I'm sure that's where I am. Yes, that has to be it."

"Uh-huh. Okay. You absolutely sure?" the voice had a condescending tone that Annabelle didn't like.

"Of course," Annabelle tried to sound haughty but instead her voice cracked with uncertainty.

The dispatcher told her that the cab would arrive in approximately ten minutes. Annabelle sat on the bed to wait. She closed her eyes and pictured Aunt Myrtle. She smiled at a memory of Aunt Myrtle in her garden, swaying against a gust of wind as she hung freshly washed clothes on the line. Annabelle pictured Aunt Myrtle wearing one of her shapeless pastel dresses, tirelessly hanging yellow, red, striped and flowered garments, all of which flapped furiously against the summer wind. Annabelle wanted to run to her. She wanted to run to that memory of Aunt Myrtle to tell her that Stanley had passed away and left her all alone. Annabelle knew Aunt Myrtle would console her like a child.

She opened her eyes and looked at the address book in her hand. It was open to Aunt Myrtle's address, which startled her. It would be a good evening for a little visit. Of course, she would need to call a cab because she really would not want to drive. She saw that the first page of the address book listed only one cab company. She picked up the phone and dialed the number.

"Blue Cab," a lazy voice answered.

Annabelle gave the dispatcher her location which was written clearly on the inside cover of the address book and without pausing gave Aunt Myrtle's address as her destination.

"Ma'am, didn't you just call us? It hasn't even been fifteen minutes."

"No, I didn't. I never called you," Annabelle said.

"Ma'am, the cab is already there at your location now," the dispatcher snapped, thoroughly annoyed.

"Oh. Well, how could that be? I mean, I barely just told you the address." Annabelle was shocked that the cab had already arrived, and even more puzzled by the dispatcher's surly tone. She thanked the voice, then looked out the window, gasping when she saw the cab parked in front of her house.

Annabelle liked the cab driver instantly. She was a huge jolly woman with coffee-colored skin who talked incessantly, pausing only to throw her head back and laugh at her own banter. Her smile was massive. Annabelle admired the woman's straight white teeth and sharp brown eyes. Both her arms were covered with flashy bracelets. She had long tiny braid extensions all over her head giving her a regal appearance.

Within the first five minutes of the ride, Annabelle knew that the driver's name was Pearl, that she had been married and divorced twice, had no living children and aspired to be an opera singer. She even sang for Annabelle. And she was good. Her voice was a booming alto with a distinctive vibrato. Annabelle hummed an unidentified gospel song along with her.

"So, sister lady, you okay? Why you out an' about this time a'night?" Pearl asked as she steered the cab onto the freeway.

"What? Well, it's not so late, really. I'm just going to visit my husband's great aunt. I haven't seen her for quite some time, and well," she chuckled a little, "it is sort of impulsive of me."

"Impulsive? Yeah, you're right about that. I thought you're gonna to visit some sick somebody this late. You sure it's his great aunt? 'Bout how old a person is that? If you don't mind my askin'," Pearl said, sneaking a quick peek at Annabelle in the rearview mirror.

"How old? I suppose I don't really know. She's never told anyone. I never asked." Annabelle stared at the back of Pearl's head, marveling at the intricacy of the tiny braids.

"Uh-hmm." Pearl was quiet, as though internally refueling for another outpouring of operatic gospel singing. But she remained silent for a while, the purring of the cab's motor dominating the empty space.

"Yes, Stanley's Aunt Myrtle is quite a character. She adores our daughter, Lily. Just adores her," Annabelle said, breaking the silence after several minutes.

"You got a daughter? How nice. Where's she?" Pearl asked.

"In Austin. My daughter lives in Austin. She's in graduate school at UT." Annabelle wasn't sure this was correct, but she couldn't remember exactly what Lily had told her about what she was doing.

"What about your husband? Stanley. Where's he? He didn't want to go along with you to see his Aunt Myrtle?" Pearl asked.

"No, no, he's at home," Annabelle said as she looked out the window. There was no traffic. Hardly any cars at all. Was it a holiday? Was it a holiday, and she didn't even know about it? Maybe it was Labor Day. Did people stay home on Labor Day? "Not too many cars tonight."

"Not this time a'night," Pearl glanced at Annabelle in the rear view mirror with an expression of brazen curiosity that began to change slowly to one of pity. The look made Annabelle uncomfortable. She felt self-conscious and began brushing tiny bits of lint off her dress.

"Where are we going?" Annabelle asked. "It seems awfully far away."

"Why, we goin' to Georgetown to the address you gave me," Pearl said, watching Annabelle intently in the mirror. She decelerated, steering the cab onto the exit ramp. "We're goin' to your auntie's house, remember? We're just about there."

When Annabelle saw Aunt Myrtle's house was darkened, she was filled with apprehension. The house looked different, too. Was it the landscaping? Had it been painted? Remodeled? Annabelle wasn't sure. There was not one light on in the house. Aunt Myrtle must be ill. Did she need help? Why hadn't she called? Annabelle glanced back at Pearl as she stepped out of the cab.

"Yes, it surely is the address you gave me, sister lady. But now, don't you worry. I'm gonna wait," Pearl said as though reading Annabelle's mind.

Annabelle knocked on the door using the big brass door knocker. She considered that the knocker might be only for decoration. It was too loud. Surely Aunt Myrtle would jolt awake and answer the door. Annabelle waited. She counted aloud to ten, then knocked again. This time she knocked more gently.

Annabelle looked around. On either side of the door there were red geranium plants in large terra-cotta pots illuminated by the amber porch light. Other unidentifiable green plants and flowers filled the rest of the porch where the aviary had once been. What had happened to all the doves and finches, Annabelle wondered. A decorative wooden bench was nearly obscured by trails of leaves and pottery, but not a trace of birds. Not the greeting sound of cooing doves or chirping finches or the odor of seed mixed with droppings. Just the silence of plants.

Annabelle was seized by a memory of Aunt Myrtle sending arm loads of potted plants home with her one Easter. The plants had been well nurtured, but after a few weeks with Annabelle, most had withered and perished.

Annabelle counted to ten again. She grabbed hold of the brass knocker but stopped abruptly when she heard footsteps. A light was switched on in the foyer. The door opened slightly.

"Yes?" It was a man. A young man of about thirty, rubbing his eyes furiously against the porch light. "What do you want?"

"I'm looking for Myrtle Storm," Annabelle said, assuming this must be a young nephew she didn't know about. She tried to look past him, but the house was dark and the door was only open enough for her to see his face and that he was wearing pajamas, which seemed odd to her. Was he sick, too?

"Who? You're looking for who?" the man said, more alert now.

"Aunt Myrtle. I'm Annabelle Storm. Stanley's wife. Is she not well?" Annabelle said, becoming more worried as she tried to look past the young man who blocked her view into Aunt Myrtle's world.

"Nobody here by that name. You must have the wrong address," answered the man. He opened the door a few more inches and looked at Annabelle with greater scrutiny. He glanced past her, noticing the taxi.

"No. No, I don't. It's right here." Annabelle thrust the address book open to Aunt Myrtle's name at him. Dull panic began to rise within her. He didn't even look at the address. He was beginning to shift uneasily.

"Look, there is no one by that name living here. This is my house. You and your address book are mistaken. Now, if you don't mind..." He started to shut the door, but Annabelle reflexively grabbed hold of it.

"Something's happened to her. Where is she? And where are the birds? Please. Tell me," Annabelle's voice began to falter.

"Birds? What're you, nuts? You're in the wrong place. I don't know who Myrtle Storm is. I've lived here for the past twelve years. This is my home. I'm going to suggest you leave before I call the police," the man said, his voice rising to anger.

"The police? Maybe I should be the one calling the police," Annabelle screamed as the door slammed abruptly in her face. She stood staring at the closed door, at the cold brass knocker and the doormat that said *Welcome Friends*. The porch light was switched off, and everything went black.

Annabelle listened to her own breathing in the darkness. It sounded jagged, unfamiliar, as though someone had stepped in to breathe in her place. The potted geraniums loomed like leafy shadows reaching for her. Suddenly she felt someone's breath on the back of her neck. She froze. A large calloused hand grabbed her arm. Her blood turned cold. She swung around, preparing to defend herself. It was Pearl.

"He's done something to her. Something dreadful— she's not—" Annabelle blurted in a whisper. She felt unbearably helpless.

"C'mon sister lady. Your auntie isn't here. We better go," Pearl said quietly. She took Annabelle by the arm and led her back to the cab.

Annabelle looked out the back window of the cab at Aunt Myrtle's house as Pearl pulled away from the curb. The house was dark again. She tried to imagine what could have happened to Aunt Myrtle and how so much time could have elapsed. A small voice within her told her that the man was lying, that he knew exactly where Stanley's aunt was. Perhaps he had caused her harm. What would she ever tell Stanley? Annabelle wondered if she should call the police after all. She noticed that Pearl kept glancing at her in the rear view mirror but said nothing.

"Wanna go on back home, sister lady?" Pearl finally asked.

"No. No, could you just drive around for a while? I have to think." Annabelle felt lost, disrupted. She was grateful for Pearl with all her tiny braids and bracelets. And kindness. Were cab drivers always this kind?

"Sure thing," Pearl said.

"Or maybe, maybe I should go see Lily. I can't remember the last time I saw my daughter," Annabelle said.

"You got her address?" Pearl asked. "Might be a real good idea."

Annabelle read Lily's address to Pearl. She sighed, then closed her eyes. There was a vacancy beginning to burrow its way into her soul. She felt powerless to stop it.

"Gonna take a while, sister lady. This here address is clear on the other side of Austin." Pearl let a low whistle escape her lips, which were pursed in thought.

"Okay. It's okay, I mean, let's just go," Annabelle said, letting her head rest on the back of the seat. She was hungry and tired. So tired.

It seemed as though only minutes had passed when the cab came to a halt. Annabelle opened her eyes wide, startled to see Pearl turned completely around staring at her. Pearl's face, which was poorly illuminated from behind by the dashboard light, was contorted with worry. It was framed by a million tiny erratic braids, making her appear mad, almost menacing. Annabelle shuddered. She realized that Pearl was speaking to her in a soft, careful voice that seemed eerie, but then somehow comical.

"What? What? Sorry, I must have dozed off," Annabelle said, stifling a laugh. She sat up straight in the seat. Where were they?

"Sister lady, we're here. We're here at your daughter's house." Pearl spoke to her like she was a small child just waking up from a nap.

"Oh, really? My daughter? How nice. Oh no, but look, her house is dark. I think that's her car in the driveway. She must be home, but her house is all dark," said Annabelle, forlorn, disappointed. With her hand on the car door handle, she turned to Pearl and asked, "You'll wait?"

"Surely will. Now you go on. Want me to go with you?" Pearl said.

"No, it's okay."

Annabelle noticed that Lily's front porch was similar to Aunt Myrtle's except that the pottery was larger, more earthy looking and arranged neatly to make room for a woven hammock filled with books. She picked up one of the books. It was a collection of T.S. Eliot's poems. She smiled at this. Her daughter had always loved poetry. Even as a small child she was captivated by any bit of prose or rhyme.

She rang the doorbell, but then decided to knock. The house was so silent. Surely Lily hadn't gone to bed early. Weren't they supposed to be having dinner together? She'd been expecting Lily for hours. Wasn't it just like Lily to become preoccupied with some lofty task and forget her own mother. Annabelle began to pound on the door, suddenly irritated.

There was a sound of footsteps, door locks being unlatched, then the door being opened slowly. Lily appeared at the entrance, sleepy eyed, dressed in shorts and an oversized T-shirt. She wore flip-flops on her feet and her hair was a chaotic mess of runaway strands.

"Mother? What are you doing here? Couldn't you sleep? Did you have a nightmare?" Lily asked as she took Annabelle by the arm and coaxed her into the house.

"Lily, really. We were supposed to be having dinner, remember? Look at you. You forgot, didn't you?" Annabelle said, clicking her tongue in disapproval.

"What are you talking about? Mother, it's 3:30 in the morning. And you're in your bathrobe. Besides we did have supper together at seven o'clock last night. At your house. I told you I'd be back this morning," Lily said, holding Annabelle at arm's length. "You're wearing your nightgown. With shoes. Tennis shoes."

"Oh good heavens, we did not either have supper at seven," Annabelle said, looking down at her bathrobe. It was her bathrobe. It seemed like a dress, but it was her bathrobe. She pulled it closer to her.

"How did you get here?" Lily asked, moving to the window to look out. "You took a cab? Is the cab waiting? Mother?"

"Cab? Oh yes. It's Pearl. She's very nice. She's waiting for me," Annabelle said

"Pearl. Well, has the cab fare been paid?" Lily asked.

"Cab fare? What?" Annabelle looked at Lily wide-eyed.

"Oh no," Lily groaned. "Mother, let me see about the cab. I'll take you home, or if you want you can stay here." Not waiting for an answer, Lily walked out to the cab with Annabelle following several tentative steps behind. Annabelle waved happily at Pearl.

"What does she owe you?" Lily dipped her head low enough to be eye to eye with Pearl who made no attempt at friendliness.

"Hundred an' three dollars," Pearl said flatly.

"What? One hundred and—" Lily gasped. She turned to look at Annabelle.

"Went to north Georgetown from northwest Austin, then from Georgetown to southwest Austin." Pearl was watching Annabelle carefully as though she might be trying to read her thoughts. "Your mama was determined to visit her Aunt Myrtle in Georgetown."

"Her Aunt Myrtle? Myrtle's been dead for years. What could she have been thinking?" Lily asked Pearl, not expecting an answer. She glanced again at Annabelle, who pretended to be unconcerned.

"She was thinkin' that she wanted to visit her auntie, that's all," Pearl snapped defensively, then added, "Lily. May I call you Lily? Your mama is real confused. Real mixed up. None of my business, but you oughta keep a close watch on her. I know something 'bout confused folks. I used to take care of a disorientated elderly lady 'fore I started drivin' this cab. Still would be, but she finally died, God bless her soul."

"Well, my dad just died a few months ago," Lily said. "Mother's been a total wreck since then. They were married for a long time."

"Uh-hmmm, I see. Yeah, that's not it," Pearl said, leveling her eyes at Lily. She glanced past Lily at Annabelle, then whispered something Annabelle couldn't quite hear.

"Of course, I'll pay for the cab ride, Lily," Annabelle said, holding up her purse, which she suddenly realized had been hanging over her shoulder since leaving her house. "Now then, how much did you say it was?"

"No, Mother, I'll pay this," Lily said wearily. "Let me go get my billfold."

She started to walk back to the house, but Pearl stopped her by shaking her head of tiny braids and holding her hands up in the air, her bracelets jangling.

"Forget it," Pearl said, "just forget about it. It's on me. I do believe that the Lord Jesus sent me to help you both tonight. You just think about what I said, Miss Lily. You think on it. Bye, bye sister lady, you promise

Pearl that you'll take care of yourself, okay? I'll be prayin' for you."

In an instant she was gone. Lily and Annabelle watched her drive away. Annabelle wondered if she should've stopped her. Pearl had been so helpful. She wondered where they had met exactly.

"Mother, really. Aunt Myrtle? Why her? You never even liked her," Lily finally said.

"Oh yes I did. She was a wonderful woman." Annabelle couldn't imagine why Lily would say such a thing.

"What happened to your thumb?" Lily took Annabelle's hand and began to examine the jagged cut along the side of her thumb with the little smears of dried blood around it. "You didn't have this cut yesterday."

"I don't know. No idea at all." Annabelle examined her thumb as if seeing it for the first time. They walked back to the house in silence.

"I'll get dressed and drive you home," Lily said. "I'll knock off from work and stay with you for a few days. How would that be? Okay?"

"Okay." Annabelle gazed up at the blackened sky. It made her sad to see the bright full moon losing its clarity to a line of gathering clouds.

*"I listened,
Threading your words
In memory,
An unselfish language"*
— *Diane Schonblom*

CHAPTER 8

Lily

"Mother, what are you doing up there?" Lily shouted from the bottom of the attic stairway.

Ten minutes earlier, Lily had Annabelle settled on the living room sofa to watch *Antique Road Show* on PBS while she went out to water the neglected garden. As the blistering sun dipped toward the horizon, Lily thought of how content Annabelle had seemed, even engrossed in what she was watching. It alarmed Lily that in such a short space of time, Annabelle had lost interest in the program and found her way up the steep staircase into the cluttered attic loft.

"I'm looking for my red suitcase," Annabelle shouted back, then added, "I just know it's here somewhere. Come help me look for it, Lily."

"Red suitcase? I thought we were looking for a red box," Lily said.

"What?" Annabelle shouted. Her voice was muffled by thousands of items stored for decades in the attic.

"Don't you mean the red box?" Lily yelled. She slumped against the wall, slid to the bottom step, then sat, holding her head in her hands.

"Red box? Box? What are you talking about? I'm looking for that old red train case." Annabelle's voice was even more muffled as she moved deeper into the endless world of storage trunks, old furniture, dusty books and neglected antiques.

"Train case? What's a train case?" Lily said without shouting. She was seized by an image of Annabelle running alongside a red caboose as it shot its way along the train track. She imagined Annabelle flailing her arms at the train to stop so she could retrieve her luggage, while the waving, smiling conductor looked straight ahead out the window, never once seeing Annabelle.

Suddenly there was a loud crash from deep in the attic.

"I'm okay," Annabelle shouted, "I didn't fall."

"Okay, Mother," Lily sighed, "I'm coming up."

She paused at the base of the staircase. A shaft of dusty sunlight from a tiny dormer window illuminated the top stairs making them appear almost like celestial steps. The attic was actually more of a spacious loft that had been partially converted into a living space.

At the top of the stairs was a small finished room, complete with a desk and small sofa next to the dormer window overlooking the flower garden. No one had ever occupied this space as far as Lily knew, but she thought perhaps her father had intended to use it as a study in his younger years. An abnormally small door at the other end of the room led to the storage area. She had to duck to pass through the door, pausing to adjust her eyes to the pale lighting of the inner attic.

It occurred to Lily that her days were spent chasing Annabelle now. She tried to stay a step ahead of her mother who teetered on the edge of instability. When they'd returned from the taxi cab fiasco, Lily was stunned to find every light on in Annabelle's house. She was horrified to discover that the dog had thrown up pear slices and rice all over the living room and that there were droplets of dried blood dotting the kitchen counter next to a hammer and a large nail. Next to the nail she found the partially eaten can of pears with its jagged lid pulled back, jutting out like sharp teeth.

And then there was the dining room table, which was lavishly set for twelve with the best china and crystal. The silverware had been placed upside down. In some cases there were only spoons. Salad bowls occupied the space for dinner plates and crystal goblets sat inside dessert saucers. There were other things, too. A kind of nonspecific disarray to the whole house, as though it were being lived in by a crazy person. Or by a child. A small undisciplined child.

A forty-watt bulb lightened the attic to a tolerable degree of dimness. The air was almost too hot to breathe. Lily brushed a cobweb off her face and shuddered. She tripped over an irregular shaped box, balancing herself against the uniform stack above it. Most of the boxes were neatly labeled. Except that, Lily noticed, almost all of the labels identified the contents as "miscellaneous things." She was surrounded by stacks and stacks of miscellaneous things. The musty smell of cardboard boxes and old wooden furniture baking in the attic heat overwhelmed her for a moment.

"Mother, are you okay?" Lily hastened her progress past an old dresser with drawers that stuck out shamelessly. She saw Annabelle sitting on the floor, her back against an old music box. She seemed suspended in time.

"Oh, good. You're here," Annabelle said, turning to look at Lily, suddenly becoming businesslike.

"You fell, didn't you?" Lily asked. She already knew the answer.

"Possibly did," Annabelle said.

"Okay. Which is it? You did or you didn't?" Lily demanded, cringing inwardly at the harshness of her own voice. She sounded like a young Annabelle interrogating

Lily as a child. She even had her hands planted firmly
on her hips, her head tipped to one side.

It was too hot. The attic air was stifling. She was
beginning to sweat. It made her angry.

To Lily's surprise, Annabelle began to cry. At first
it was a sniffle. Then tears began to roll down her face.
Lily stared at her mother. It unnerved her to see Annabelle sitting in a heap on the attic floor, whimpering
like a small child. Rarely had she seen Annabelle give
way to emotion. Annabelle had always been so decisive,
so absurdly organized and always intolerant of any
perceived weakness in Lily.

"You shouldn't have been up here rummaging around
in all this mess." Lily felt detached from her own voice,
as though it came from some part of her that had been
horribly hurt by her mother and now wanted her to pay
for the pain. "You're injured, aren't you?" she added
more softly.

"No--I'm fine. Didn't I tell you that already? Don't
you listen? You want me to be hurt, don't you? Is that
it? You just want me to be hurt?" Annabelle snapped as
she blotted her eyes with a crumpled tissue. She touched
her injured wrist and winced, suddenly belting out a
shrill stream of profanities.

Lily was taken aback. Hearing Annabelle curse
was like being slapped sharply across the face by Betty
Crocker. Her first instinct was to turn and walk away. Let
Annabelle figure her way out of her own mess. That's
exactly what Annabelle would have done to Lily. And,
she had done that. When Lily had a vulnerable moment,
Annabelle had always insisted that Lily be strong, not
give in to emotion, and then, Annabelle would simply
walk away, making no attempt to reassure her.

Stanley had been the one to provide the comfort,
telling Lily that yes, your mother does care about you.
She cares more than you could imagine—she just has
a different way of showing it. She just wants you to be

strong enough for the world, Lily, he would say. She doesn't want emotion to cloud your judgment and plus, he would add, life had not always been easy for Annabelle.

Lily hovered between the memory of her father's words and of Annabelle sitting on the attic floor in front of her. Something inside her froze. Her limbs were paralyzed. She was unable to reach out to Annabelle.

"I may have broken my wrist," Annabelle said in a sullen voice. She produced a swollen, discolored left hand. She gazed up at Lily, blinking back tears.

Finally Lily sank to the floor in front of Annabelle. She sat cross-legged and gently took Annabelle's outstretched hand. It looked distorted and painful. There were no objects near Annabelle, as far as Lily could see, that could have caused such an injury. It must have been the fall. Annabelle must have tried to break her fall.

"I'm sorry. I'm sorry I did this. I don't know how I got up here to the attic. I just thought—" Annabelle words floated away. She looked down at her hand.

"Well, we'd better get you to the hospital," Lily said. Annabelle's apology made Lily even more uneasy. It seemed out of place. Where was the old Annabelle who would have jumped up and regained her composure? Was Stanley's absence causing Annabelle to lose her hard exterior?

Suddenly Lily wanted to shake her mother. She wanted the familiar Annabelle back. The critical, flawless Annabelle. Why, so many years later, when it was just too late, did Lily have to discover that her mother had a fragile side, that she could feel remorse, that she could be careless enough to break her wrist?

Annabelle began to swear. Sweat beads trickled down her forehead into her eyes, dropping off her nose.

"Why are you cursing all of a sudden?" Lily let go of her mother's hand too abruptly.

"I don't know. It hurts. My whole arm hurts." Annabelle continued shouting, "Just help me up! NOW!"

"You have got to stop this insane search for that red box, Mother. I don't know what's in it and why you're obsessing over it, but it's just got to stop," Lily said as she helped Annabelle to her feet. "At least wait until I can help you. I just cannot imagine what could be so important—"

"It's in Minnesota. I just know it is. At the lake cottage. We really ought to go there, Lily. Couldn't we go right away?" Annabelle's tone was earnest, almost whining, like a child trying to talk a parent into something forbidden.

"But we just got back from the lake cottage —oh god, never mind," Lily said. The back of her T-shirt, dampened with perspiration, now stuck to her skin. She desperately needed to breathe cooled air.

The emergency room was crowded with blubbering kids and glassy-eyed adults. Everyone seemed horribly ill. Lily settled Annabelle in one of the hard cushioned chairs, then walked to the admissions desk. She glanced back at Annabelle who looked as blank as the wall behind her. Annabelle had insisted on bringing her purse, but then had handed it over to Lily after she was seated as though it meant nothing to her. As though it was some annoying object she'd found on the floor.

The wait to see a doctor was shorter than Lily would have anticipated. The doctor was a young, curly haired man with black rimmed glasses who made poor eye contact. He seemed nervous and ready to spring off into another direction at any given moment.

"We'll get an x-ray, but yeah, there's a definite fracture here," he said. "Does your mother have any other health problems?"

She's right here, ask her yourself, Lily wanted to say, but found herself telling him that she wasn't actually sure. When he asked about medications or allergies, Lily automatically opened Annabelle's purse. She gasped slightly when she saw what seemed like an endless supply of prescription bottles.

"I guess these are her medicines," Lily placed the bottles on the little desk in front of her. Suddenly she felt ashamed that she knew so little about Annabelle's health. The doctor was looking at her directly now, as though he sensed her guilt.

He looked at each bottle briefly, making little notes on the chart in front of him. When he was finished, he turned to face Annabelle and smiled at her. Annabelle smiled back wearily.

"Mrs. Storm, are you allergic to anything?" he asked.

"I don't like cucumbers," Annabelle said.

"Me neither," the doctor chuckled. He turned to look at Lily.

"I really have no idea about her allergies. Is it important? I know who her regular doctor is. Would that help?" Lily said.

"So," the doctor said, ignoring her question. He looked back at the chart. "How exactly did this happen?"

"She fell," Lily answered.

"Fell," he repeated, stroking his chin thoughtfully.

"She was looking for something in our attic. I didn't actually see her fall." Lily wondered if the doctor suspected her of elder abuse. The thought of it made her furious.

"How long has Mrs. Storm had Alzheimer's disease?" The doctor fixed his gaze on Annabelle who was brushing invisible lint off her blouse.

"Alzheimer's? What? My mother does not have Alzheimer's disease! What would make you say such a thing? Look at her chart, she's only fifty-two!" Lily shouted. Then lowering her voice added, "My mother fell. She tried to break her fall. She broke her wrist. What kind of doctor are you? How do you get Alzheimer's out of that?"

"Her medicines," the doctor answered simply, unfazed by Lily's outburst. "Namenda, Aricept, Risperdal. These are drugs commonly prescribed for patients with Alzheimer's."

Lily looked from the doctor to Annabelle. She opened her mouth to speak, but the words wouldn't come. At that moment, she was struck by the sheer emptiness of Annabelle's expression. She was struck by the fact that Annabelle didn't spring to her feet and tell the doctor how wrong he was.

"She also takes cardiac medicines and a blood thinner," he continued, ignoring Lily's inability to speak. "Who takes care of your mother?"

"She does. I mean, my dad did. Well, it's her—but then, I guess—me. I do. I mean, it's me. I'm taking care of her. But she has been—" Lily stammered.

"You're taking care of her, but you didn't know she has Alzheimer's?" The doctor looked over the rim of his glasses at Lily, then sat back in his chair, which rolled slightly against the shift in weight.

"My dad just died two months ago. He always took care of Mother," Lily said defensively.

"And you're saying that he never told you about her illness?" The doctor drummed his fingers on the desk, knocking one of the medicine bottles over.

"That's right," Lily answered glumly. She felt miserable.

All of a sudden the doctor sprang to his feet, picked up Annabelle's chart and walked to the edge of the exam cubicle. He opened the privacy curtain enough to summon a nurse, then turned back to Lily.

"We'll get an x-ray, immobilize her wrist. Then she's free to go," he said. "I would suggest that you get with her doctor first thing tomorrow to come up with a plan to keep your mother safe."

The curtain swished behind him as he strolled away. Lily stared at the curtain until it stopped moving. She turned to look at Annabelle who was putting the medicine bottles back in her purse. Lily had no idea what to say to her mother.

"Can we go home now?" Annabelle asked.

"No, Mother, you have to get your hand and wrist x-rayed. Then they're going to put a splint or a cast on it," Lily answered, suddenly realizing she was speaking in an exaggerated voice, forming each word carefully as though this were the only way her mother would understand her.

"What happened to my wrist?" Annabelle asked in a booming voice, enunciating her words the same exaggerated way Lily had just done.

"You fractured your wrist when you fell in the attic, Mother," Lily said.

"Is Stanley coming?"

"No, Mother, Dad passed away in April," Lily answered, wondering if this was the right thing to say. Wouldn't it be easier just to say yes? *Yes, Mother, Dad will be here soon, he's just parking the car.*

"Oh no, oh no. That's right. Oh, poor Stanley," Annabelle said softly as she put her good hand to her face. She closed her eyes and sighed deeply.

They spoke very little while Annabelle's wrist was x-rayed and splinted. They spoke even less on the car trip home. Lily felt as though her head would burst with questions she knew Annabelle couldn't answer. Had Annabelle remembered to take her medicine regularly? How long had Annabelle had this horrid disease? Why, why, why had Stanley not told her that her mother had Alzheimer's? How long had he been protecting Annabelle from the world? And from her? What was she supposed to do about her mother now? Had her father thought he could just take care of Annabelle forever?

And then, Lily was angry. Fury boiled inside her as she thought of what her father had left behind. He'd left her to coexist with Annabelle, yes. But this was even worse because he'd left her to coexist with a broken version of her mother. And with no warning. She wanted to shake her fist at heaven, tell him to come back and fix this.

Lily glanced at her mother. She was there—right there, sitting beside Lily in the car, looking straight ahead at the road. Her face was vacant. She said nothing. Annabelle was gone, or going away, she was leaving Lily. It was as though Annabelle had been defeated when the word Alzheimer's was said out loud. Lily wondered how much Annabelle understood. Did she know her mind was failing?

"I don't want this," Annabelle said suddenly, breaking Lily's thoughts apart. She tugged at the splint on her left arm.

"No! No, you have to keep that on, don't do that," Lily almost shouted.

Annabelle stopped tugging and looked at Lily. Her expression was a contorted mixture of shock and annoyance.

"The doctor prescribed some pain pills, Mother. I'll give you one when we get back to the house," Lily said.

"Oh no, I do not take medicine," Annabelle answered firmly.

"It will help with the pain, Mother." Lily wondered if her father had been through this same thing.

They drove the rest of the way in heavy silence. When they arrived at Annabelle's house, Caesar greeted them in the street just as another car shot by, barely missing the dog.

"Oh my god, what is Caesar doing out here?" Lily slammed the car into park and jumped out to retrieve the dog. Once she had him, it dawned on her that the poor dog was skin and bones. Annabelle could no more take care of her favorite canine companion than she could herself. Annabelle had likely put him out the front door by mistake when they'd left for the hospital. The dog would surely die one way or another if Annabelle continued to care for him.

"It's late. You probably should get to bed, Mother," Lily said once they were inside the house. She managed to get Annabelle to swallow her pain medicine, but when she attempted the other pills Annabelle recoiled, claiming Lily was trying to poison her.

"I don't go to bed this early," Annabelle said with finality. Her eyes were puffy and reddened. She looked exhausted, and yet poised for conflict, ready to defend herself.

"Oh well, okay." Lily didn't bother telling her mother that it was already after midnight. Instead, she unfolded a quilt across the living room sofa, patted a large pillow into place at one end and said, "Maybe you could just rest right here. That is, if you want."

"Where's my dog?" Annabelle demanded. She stood in the center of the room, cradling her injured wrist, peering around her as if she were in someone else's home.

"Caesar's in the kitchen eating his dog food. He's fine. Hungry, but okay," Lily answered.

"Oh," Annabelle said, "Caesar's eating his dinner," as if telling herself.

She continued standing in the center of the room, not moving, expressionless. Finally Lily took her gently by the arm and led her to the sofa. Annabelle sat heavily, wearily, her breath coming in small puffs. Caesar trotted into the room and sat at her feet, letting out a noisy extended burp of satisfaction at having eaten his first bowl of dog food in what had likely been a very long time. Both women laughed as the dog wagged his tail happily. He put his head in Annabelle's lap. Her laughter faded abruptly. She placed her good hand on his head as her eyes brimmed with quiet tears. Lily wondered if Annabelle knew on some level that she had not been caring for her dog properly.

"See, he's fine," Lily said.

"I can't take care of him," Annabelle said unexpectedly, surprising even herself. She looked from the dog to Lily, her eyes widened with a kind of bewilderment Lily had never seen in her mother.

"It's okay, Mother. I'll do it. I'll stay here at your house for now. What do you think about that idea?" Lily said. It had occurred to her at that moment that Annabelle could never be left alone again. The thought of it filled her with a sorrow worse than grief. Lily would have to hire someone to stay with Annabelle when she was at work. But who? What sort of person would Annabelle let stay with her? It seemed like such an intrusion.

Lily let her anger at Stanley rise again for leaving behind such a mess. It just made no sense. She'd adored her father to the point of believing he could do no wrong. How was it possible that he could have let her down like this?

"No, Lily, you cannot miss school. I will not have you missing school," Annabelle was saying, sounding more like her former self. The strict, inflexible, oppressive Annabelle. And yet her voice was filled with fatigue. Her words slurred, her eyelid's drooped. The pain medicine was taking hold of her.

"School? I don't have—" Lily started to correct Annabelle but stopped herself. "I-I don't have school, uh, because it's summer. School's out for summer. So, see? Nothing to worry about."

But Annabelle had fallen asleep. Her head lolled to one side, shoulders slumped forward. She had not heard the first of many benevolent lies she would be told over the months to come. Lily went to her, took off her shoes, lifted her legs onto the sofa, and placed her head on the pillow, pulling the quilt over her. Annabelle did not awaken. Her expression was peaceful now. She had drifted into the safe, cottony world of dreams where nonsense rules.

Lily sat back in her father's deep cushioned rocking chair across from Annabelle and watched her sleep. She watched her mother breathe steadily in and out, undisturbed. The perpetual little lines of worry around her eyes and mouth had faded into soft slumber. And all Lily could think was, *Alzheimer's*. Alzheimer's disease. My mother is going to lose her mind.

She tried to recall what she knew about the disease, concluding only that it had something to do with deterioration of the brain affecting memory, that there was no cure, and that it was a cruel, heartless thief of self. A thief who would eventually steal away a mother she had never really known.

At two o'clock in the morning, Lily decided to return to the attic loft. It was useless trying to sleep. Something about Annabelle's fall kept nagging at her. Her mother was still agile, even light footed, like a dancer. What had made her lose her balance? What had caught her attention enough to cause her to be so careless? Vaguely, Lily remembered seeing a book on the floor next to her mother. And a key. Some sort of ancient-looking key. She glanced back at Annabelle on the sofa, who was now snoring in harmony with Caesar.

Lily retraced her footsteps from the evening before into the attic, ducking into the entrance and wiping another cobweb from her face. Even with the light on, the room was as dim as candlelight. And there was that nauseating smell of old furniture, mildew and cardboard.

Lily was again intrigued by the number of boxes her parents had labeled as miscellaneous *items*. Why even label them, she wondered. She was struck by the thought that it would eventually be her responsibility to sort through all the storage boxes. Maybe even soon. She cringed inwardly. The thought of sorting through all of her parents' belongings saddened her. How had this happened so quickly? It seemed only yesterday that she was just a girl hiding in this attic from one of the baby-sitters she hadn't liked.

When she reached the far end where Annabelle had fallen, she noticed that a few of the largest boxes, also labeled *miscellaneous items,* had been forced open. Old garments and linens were billowing out of one box as though someone had been frantically trying to reach the bottom.

Another box was gaping open, revealing sewing supplies, thread and button-filled baskets and dress patterns. When she reached across to look in another box, Lily stepped down onto a hard object. She looked at the floor. It was the book Annabelle had been sitting next to after her fall.

Slowly Lily picked up the book. It was large but not particularly heavy. And yet, she could see how it might have become awkward for Annabelle to maneuver the book while standing in the middle of the box contents strewn all over the floor. It was clear that Annabelle had been searching wildly for the red train case or suitcase or box without regard to the chaotic disorder she was creating all around her.

Lily sat on the floor in the same spot where Annabelle had fallen. She opened the book. It was an old photo album filled with photos Lily had never seen before. There were baby pictures of Annabelle's parents that were so tattered and yellowed Lily avoided touching or even breathing on them. Their wedding photo, which was a little better preserved, was on the same page. Someone had written, *Mr. and Mrs. Noble Doyle* across the bottom of the photo. Lily thought the couple looked too somber for newlyweds. Annabelle's mother was wearing a starched looking dress that covered her entire body except for her face and hands. Lily imagined that her grandmother had had to be carried in and out of her wedding like a large wooden doll.

The next pages were filled with baby and childhood photos of Annabelle. Lily was fascinated with how happy her mother looked. In almost every picture, she was smiling, even laughing, her little face beaming with joy. Or no, not joy. More like mischief. Her mother looked very impish. In one family photo, Annabelle's parents seemed stern, unforgiving, but there was little Annabelle in the foreground, carefree and smiling ear to ear.

It was the next section of photos that made Lily stand up so that she could be closer to the overhead light. She sucked in a deep breath. There was Annabelle as a young girl, as a teenager, and as a young woman staring at her from across the years with a smile that had changed from impish to daring. Something in the way she tipped her head, the way she placed one hand on her hip made her appear impudent, unruly. There were dozens and dozens of photos of Annabelle in her late teens. Lily was amazed at how reckless her mother appeared.

There was an enlargement of the only early photo Lily had ever seen of her mother. It was a candid photo of Annabelle in Minnesota standing at the edge of the dock, wind gusts threatening to throw her off balance. She had one hand on her hip and the other shielding her eyes, scanning the horizon, searching for something.

"What were you looking for, Mother?" Lily said aloud. To Lily, the photo represented everything she didn't know about her mother. It made her feel desperate and a little lonely. Who was this woman who became her mother?

The pages that followed were filled with photos of houses, flowers gardens in black and white, a few of someone's prize Tennessee Walker. There seemed to be some sequence to it all. Lily thumbed through the pages with only mild interest until she came upon a page of photos of two older teenage boys. The boys were both handsome in a careless James Dean sort of way. Cigarettes dangled from their mouths. They wore leather jackets and jeans. They were leaning against a motorcycle. There were several more pages of the two boys. Lily was struck by their good looks, their wild, windblown hair and tanned faces.

And then it hit her. One of the two boys was Frankie as a teenager. Frankie, the man from the grocery store in Minnesota. Frankie, who had called Annabelle, *Annabelle Doyle*. Frankie, who Annabelle said she didn't remember. She had said that maybe Frankie wasn't even his real name. Frankie, who had only a six pack of beer and a loaf of bread in his shopping cart, and had commented about how much Lily looked like Annabelle.

It was definitely the same person. But how was it possible that Annabelle did not remember him? On the next page, there she was, the daring, defiant young Annabelle barefoot and wearing shorts over a swimsuit, sitting on the hood of an old Ford convertible with Frankie and the other handsome boy. Except that she was sitting closer to the other boy. He had his arm around her shoulders, and they were laughing carelessly.

And then, the photo album ended abruptly. There were no pictures of Stanley, no wedding photos or photos of Lily as a baby. Instead there were blank pages, never to be filled. Lily felt an emptiness in the pit of her stomach. She sat on the floor and studied each photo again.

There was only so much to be learned from old photos. The only photo that had identification was the wedding photo of Mr. and Mrs. Noble Doyle. Lily's grandparents. People she never really knew. She vaguely remembered that they'd died less than a week apart and that Annabelle had quietly left Texas for their funerals in South Dakota, saying very little upon her return. She hadn't even seemed sad. A bit preoccupied, but not sad.

Lily sighed heavily. She had only had a glimpse into Annabelle's childhood. It was like looking into the tiny window of a doll house. Nothing more. Stanley had always told her that Annabelle's life had been hard but had declined to elaborate when Lily pressed him for details. He would tell her that it was up to Annabelle to tell Lily what she wanted her to know. But Annabelle had never talked about her earlier years. Lily had grown accustomed to not asking. It had become nearly unimportant.

Lily closed her eyes and leaned back against the box of sewing supplies. Suddenly she felt unbearably alone. Had Annabelle intended for her to find this photo album? But why? And had she been crying because her wrist hurt or was she crying because she had been looking at the photos of her youth? Or was it just more of Annabelle's recent erratic behavior?

The word Alzheimer's bored its way into her thoughts again. Alzheimer's. How long? How long had Annabelle had this? She was too young for this. Far too young. There must be some mistake. Was this early onset version of the illness hereditary?

Early the next morning Lily stood in the kitchen with her hand on the phone, intending to call Annabelle's doctor. She could see from the kitchen door that Annabelle was still sleeping soundly in the living room. Caesar had climbed onto the sofa with her, and the two of them lay there peacefully in a swirl of covers and pillows. Lily watched them for a moment, then picked up the phone and punched in Tess's number. She felt a new desperation to talk with someone who had known her mother before all this. Someone who could understand how baffling it was to contemplate a deteriorating Annabelle.

Teddy answered the call, telling Lily that Tess was at the Gray Dawn having an early breakfast with someone. He was vague and preoccupied, but polite as usual. Lily dialed the number for the Gray Dawn Café.

"Gray Dawn," Will Larson sounded almost too cheery. Lily wanted to hang up.

"Will. It's Lily. How are you?" Lily asked.

"Oh, hey, this is a surprise. I'm good, what about you? How are things in Texas?"

"Okay, I guess. It's Mother. She's having a tough time." Lily wanted to unload every sad detail, let him try to make her feel better. He seemed like that kind of guy. The guy who would listen to every detail, then have something comforting and reasonable to say that would make it all better. "Can I talk to Tess? Is she there? It's important."

"Oh yeah, sure. She's right here," Will said. Lily could hear him tell Tess that the call was important.

"Lily. Are you okay? What is it?" Tess wasted no time on pleasantries.

"You were right, Tess. Mother has Alzheimer's disease," Lily blurted, shrinking into her own words, waiting for Tess to tell her she was wrong.

"Oh no! Oh Lily. How is that even possible—she's too young."

"It's that early onset Alzheimer's, I guess. Probably she's had it for a long time."

"I am so sorry. I knew something wasn't right. Did you have to take her to the doctor? What happened?" Tess said.

"I had to take her to the emergency room last night. She broke her wrist looking for that stupid red box in the attic. The ER doctor looked at her prescription bottles and told me about the Alzheimer's, but I just couldn't—you know—it was so—I still can't quite—," Lily's words vanished into air. She stopped trying to talk.

"How awful, Lily. Are you okay? When could she have been diagnosed with it? Why had no one told you? Your dad, didn't he—" Tess started.

"Dad had to have known. He just never told me. He never told me, Tess, " Lily repeated mechanically. "Dad never told me."

Neither of them spoke for a moment. Lily silently reviewed her mother's behavior over the last year, the last two years, the last five. In each memory, her father loomed in the foreground, a protective shadow over his failing wife.

"Well, what are you going to do? Is there something I can do?" Tess sounded smaller and less confident.

"I don't know. But Tess, there's something else. I found an old photo album in the attic. There were pictures of Annabelle when she was in her late teens and pictures of two teenage boys. Well, young men, really. A lot of photos of them. They seemed sort of like, uh, I don't know, James Dean. You know, bad boys. I recognized one of them from someone we saw at the grocery store in town. His name was Frankie. He knew Annabelle, but she wanted nothing to do with him. Do you know him?" Lily asked.

"Frankie? No, no, I really don't. This town is small, but not that small. I don't know any grown men with the name Frankie. Unless, wait. There's that guy who works at the hardware store in the summer. Could be him. I think his name is Frank, though," Tess said, adding, "Lily, why is this important? What are you going to do about Annabelle?"

"I know I'm not putting her in one of those homes. I know that. I'll find a way to take care of her," Lily said forcefully.

"Okay. But what about you, Lily? What about your job—your garden shop?" Tess sounded motherly and slightly scolding.

"I don't know. I just don't know anything. I'll talk to her doctor. I'll find someone to come in and stay with her while I'm at work, I guess," Lily said.

"But for how long? Will Annabelle be okay with a stranger in the house? I don't know, Lily. Your mom is so private and I mean, almost secretive. And so strict about everything," Tess said. "Do you want me to come down there for a while? I can."

"No, Tess. No, no, it'll be okay," Lily wanted to say yes. *Yes, Tess, please come help me with this. I'm so afraid I'm going to get this whole thing wrong. I'll disappoint Annabelle somehow. I won't measure up, won't do things correctly. This is my last chance to get things right with my mother.*

Lily wasted no time calling the doctor's office after she and Tess said good-bye. The receptionist put her through to the nurse who put her on hold again to go talk with the doctor. While Lily waited, she opened the cupboard in front of her. Her hand flew to her mouth as she gasped aloud. The cupboard was packed from top to bottom with Girl Scout cookies. There was nothing else. Just cookies. There must have been over thirty boxes, all unopened.

The doctor's office hold music shifted to a dramatic, crashing classical piece making the discovery of the cookies feel like the beginning of a choreographed drama. She opened another cupboard. In it, she found three unmatched socks, a dried partially eaten bowl of oatmeal with a spoon stuck to the side, an empty box of Uncle Ben's rice, a tennis shoe, two slices of molded bread, raisins in an envelop from the bank and a broken glass framed photo of Lily when she was eight. She quickly shut the cupboard door.

"Dr. Mason wants to know if you and Mrs. Storm can come in this afternoon at two o'clock," the nurse was saying.

"Okay, we'll be there," Lily answered grimly.

"Again, I'm so sorry about Mr. Storm. We didn't know. He was such a wonderful man. Really took good care of Mrs. Storm," the nurse said.

Dr. Mason was a kindly older gentleman who seemed to care deeply about his patients. He was short and round and balding. He wore thick glasses, which he had a habit of removing continually to rub his eyes. Annabelle was utterly at ease in his presence. He spoke with her in a light conversational way, never wavering when her side of the conversation made no sense. He had his nurse take Annabelle off to the lab for blood tests, then motioned for Lily to sit in the chair across from him.

"So, I take it your dad didn't tell you about the Alzheimer's?" he asked.

"He never said anything," Lily was grateful to finally be talking to someone who knew something. "Isn't she awfully young?"

"She's young all right, but it happens. Early onset. Lily, your mother was diagnosed with Alzheimer's disease several years ago." Dr. Mason studied her.

"No, wait. How is that possible? My dad never—but he always—and she never even…" Lily's voice trailed off. "How do you know? I mean, was she tested for it? When did this happen?"

Dr. Mason stood up. Yellow sunlight sliced through a nearby window blind, falling in stripes across his lab coat as he turned his back to her. He sunk both hands into his pockets and began to jangle change. The tinkling sound of loose coins filled the momentary silence. He took off his glasses and rubbed his eyes with his thumb.

"I'm so sorry Stanley never told you about this. Hell of a way to find out. Your dad was a wonderful human being. Probably thought he was protecting her somehow. Chances are he'd planned to tell you when things got too bad," he said, turning back to Lily. "I sent your mother to a neurologist. He made the diagnosis."

Lily said nothing. So, it was true. Annabelle had this dreaded illness, and she eventually would fade away. Dr. Mason watched Lily intently as she absorbed the reality of it.

"She has had episodes of extreme erratic behavior. Your dad must have worked very hard keeping it a secret. The medicines helped some. Especially with her uncontrolled rage," Dr. Mason said.

"Uncontrolled rage? Erratic behavior? Dr. Mason, I'm fairly certain my mother hasn't been taking her medicines since Dad died," Lily said.

"Hmmm. That's not good. What about incontinence?" he asked suddenly.

"Incontin—what?" Lily asked.

"I mean is she able to make it to the bathroom okay?"

"I guess. I guess so. I'm not completely sure. Oh no, no, I'm sure she doesn't have that. She gets to the bathroom just fine. I would have noticed during the time we were in Minnesota after Dad died," Lily said.

"What about wandering? Wandering away from the house?"

"No," Lily answered, thinking of Annabelle's taxi ride with Pearl, wondering if that counted as wandering.

"She's dressing herself okay?"

"Oh, yes, I believe so." Lily remembered when Annabelle had her slippers or shoes on the wrong feet. And the time she stood on Tess and Sam's dock in her socks with no coat against the bitter cold. Was that important?

"Falls? Any other falls?" he asked.

"No," Lily answered, but the truth was, she didn't know. She shifted uneasily in her chair as she watched Dr. Mason move to stand behind his. He placed both hands on the back of the chair and began smoothing its surface. He gazed pensively up at the ceiling as though their entire conversation had been documented there.

"She can't be left alone, Lily. You do realize that, don't you?" the doctor said. He sat heavily in his chair, picked up Annabelle's chart and leveled his gaze at Lily. "Her weight has dropped significantly, her blood pressure is up; she's terribly confused, anxious. She can't take care of herself." He paused. "You might want to think about placing her in a facility tailored for her type of dementia."

"What? Oh god, no. I couldn't do that," Lily said. "That's probably what Dad was afraid of more than anything. I hate those places. I mean, I guess I hate those places. I've never really had any experience."

Dr. Mason frowned, removed his glasses slowly, then began to rub his eyes for the hundredth time as if he was terribly weary. As though rubbing his eyes would somehow clear the problem in front of him. Lily noticed a spot on his chin that he had missed shaving. It distracted her because the man seemed so articulate. It made him suddenly seem less believable.

"I'll hire someone, and I'll move in with her for the time being. Or something," Lily said. "She won't be left alone. Ever."

"I can give you the names of some local agencies that employ unskilled caretakers, if you like," he said, "but eventually she's going to need something more. She'll need nurses, Lily. Your mother has other health problems, too. I'm going to give you a detailed list of her medications. I want to see her back here in a month."

"Okay," Lily said.

"She can't drive, you know. Very dangerous. She almost ran over her neighbor's little girl last year," Dr. Mason said. "Your dad wouldn't have told you, but she also drove to southeast Austin, then called him on a pay phone, totally lost, not able to tell him where she was or even describe what was around her. With great effort, your dad convinced her go to a police officer for help. She was gone a total of ten hours. Very harrowing experience."

"My god, I didn't know any of this," Lily said, then added carefully, "Dr. Mason, my mother and I, we've, well, we've never gotten along all that well. She tends to oppose most everything I tell her. It's as though I'm her unruly teenage daughter who she has to set straight. I was never unruly. Not really."

"Lily, you have to let go of that. Let it go. Your mother's mind is slipping away," he said gently. "We need to go ahead and see about making arrangements for power of attorney to be changed to you. It has to be done."

In the days that followed the visit with Dr. Mason, Lily researched local home care agencies. She conducted three interviews of kindly women she felt would be well suited in caring for Annabelle while she was at work. But Annabelle became paranoid and suspicious at each interview, even openly rude to the youngest of the applicants. To Lily's horror, her mother told the young woman that she looked like a little slut, that she had no business in their house and that she needed to go straight home and get dressed. Lily was too shocked by her mother's uncharacteristic outburst to apologize. The young woman, who was dressed in an attractive sundress and sandals was immediately unnerved and cut the interview short.

Lily considered bringing Annabelle with her to work at the Green Thumb Garden Shoppe every day. She could find something for her to do, couldn't she? Something that would give Annabelle a sense of purpose. Lily could keep a steady eye on her mother and still get her work done.

The idea lasted two days. The first day Annabelle seemed to enjoy buzzing around, watering plants and greeting customers. A few times she said things that were odd, out of place, but if anyone was alarmed by this, nothing was said. She even helped the clerk reorganize a display of small cactus plants. She seemed calm and happy. Lily had slipped Annabelle's medicine into her food that morning and she had taken it without noticing. It all seemed very promising. Lily forced herself to ignore the multitude of times her mother would pop into her office and remind her she needed to come out of her room and get her chores done. Or the repetition. Annabelle continually asked Lily, the shop clerk, and the assistant manager if it was time for breakfast, or when would she be going home, or did they know where her purse was. Over and over and over.

The second day, she disappeared. In a matter of minutes, Annabelle was gone. Lily panicked. No one in the shop actually saw Annabelle leave. Lily sprinted up and down the street, asking everyone in her path if they had seen a woman with long graying hair tied into a braid down her back. She was wearing jeans, a red gingham blouse and tennis shoes. She might seem confused. She's thin. Has dark eyes and was wearing a hat. What kind of hat? A baseball cap. Yes, that was it. Annabelle had put the Green Thumb Garden Shoppe baseball cap on when she'd arrived that morning. She'd taken her medicine again. She seemed happy.

The assistant shop manager began to sprint along with Lily, peering into alleyways and storefronts. Suddenly he stopped, turned to Lily and suggested they extend their search into opposite circles.

"She couldn't have gotten that far. My god, she was only gone a minute," Lily said, agreeing to split the search. She decided to begin driving around the block while he asked the nearby shop owners if they'd seen Annabelle. There was a sandwich shop to check, a used book store, a gift shop, men's clothing store, a bakery. Lily glanced in her rearview mirror as the assistant manager disappeared into the gift shop.

Driving around the blocks proved to be futile. Lily was in a full state of panic. She ran a red light. Car horns honked furiously. She slowed down. Then she thought she saw Annabelle on the opposite side of the street, walking fast, almost running. Lily's foot hit the accelerator hard. But it wasn't Annabelle. She drove in wider circles around the next block. The next. She changed lanes sharply, cutting off the car behind her. The driver cursed, honked his horn, glared at her as he shot past. Lily slowed the car but still managed to run another red light.

When she noticed the cop car's flashing light behind her, she stopped the car so fast that she jerked forward. She jumped out and dashed toward the police officer who was barely out of his patrol car.

"Officer, you've got to help me. Please, my mother is—she left my—she has Alzheimer's and she's going to be—" the words came out in a rush. Lily felt her head swim when she said the word Alzheimer's. *My mother has Alzheimer's disease.*

"Whoa. Just wait one minute. You need to stop right there. I'm going to need to see your driver's license and proof of insurance. You just exceeded the speed limit by ten miles per hour, and you ran two red lights," the cop's manner was gruff, unyielding.

Lily felt nauseated. Her mother was getting further and further away while she was being stopped by some boy scout cop. She retrieved her purse from the car and produced her license and insurance for the policeman who spent an inordinate amount of time sitting in the front seat of his car talking into his two-way radio and making notes on a clipboard. Lily stood beside her car but continued to look up and down the street for Annabelle. She knew she likely looked suspicious to the cop by now, but she didn't care. He was making her angrier than she'd been in a long time.

"So what's this about your mother with Alzheimer's?" he said, returning her license. He had written her a ticket for running the red lights. Lily was livid.

"Well, no thanks to you, she's probably in Bastrop County by now," Lily said, getting back into her car.

"Ma'am, you ran two red lights speeding," he said defensively, his gruffness returning, "you or someone else could have been hurt."

"I know, I know," Lily groaned. She put her head in her hands and took a long deep breath. This cop was young and filled with self-importance. She looked up at him, "My mother came with me to work. I own the

Green Thumb Garden Shoppe. She has Alzheimer's. She wandered away. She could be anywhere. I have to find her. She's so confused. She's liable to—." She couldn't continue, overcome with this unwanted responsibility for a deteriorating Annabelle.

"Okay. Let's see what we can do," the cop said. He asked Lily questions. What was her mother wearing. How long had she been gone. Which way was she most likely to go. Did she know enough to ask for help. The questions were endless. Somehow Lily ended up at the police station answering even more questions. Annabelle hadn't been gone even twenty-four hours, but she was mentally disabled. It was different. More urgent. People wanted to help find her. One police officer even said he remembered Annabelle Storm from another occasion when she had wandered away from home. Lily wondered if that were true. And if it was, how had her father managed this by himself?

Lily returned home to wait. She sat in the living room with the phone in her lap, Annabelle's dog at her feet. Hours passed. Unbearable tense hours. Lily would never forgive herself for this. She had lost her own mother. What could have been in Annabelle's mind to wander away like that?

Lily remembered a time when she was ten, maybe eleven, when she herself had wandered away from her mother at a huge department store. It had happened so fast. They had been shopping for school clothes and Lily had almost convinced Annabelle to buy her one of the new shorter style skirts. When Annabelle finally found her, she had been furious, unforgiving, telling Lily that anything could have happened to her, that there were bad people in the world lying in wait for the right moment to snatch away an innocent child. She had been harsh, her face red with an inner rage and yet blanching with worry. She threw the skirts and blouses she'd been carrying onto a nearby display table and stomped out of the store, dragging Lily behind her, muttering that the skirts were too short and what could she have been thinking.

Wasn't it the same somehow? Annabelle was now the innocent one, her mind slipping away, becoming more childlike everyday. Anything could happen to her. Even bad people lying in wait for the right moment to snatch away an innocent demented woman.

The phone in her lap rang. Lily shot forward, stood up, answered.

"Your mother has been found," the police officer was saying. "She was up on IH-35 walking along the frontage road. They've taken her to the City Medical Center emergency room."

"Emergency room? What? Why? Is she hurt?" Lily said.

"They're checking her for heatstroke," he said simply, "but I'm pretty sure she's okay."

Annabelle was released nearly eight hours later in stable condition. She was exhausted and had no real recollection of what had happened. She fell asleep sitting in Stanley's old recliner chair while Lily sat fully dressed, fully awake, unblinking, watching over her mother like a personal sentry.

Something had to change. This wasn't working. Annabelle was too unpredictable. Lily spent the rest of the night considering her options, wishing her father was there to discuss it with her. She watched her mother breathe in and out, watched her eyelashes flutter, listened to her snore lightly.

When morning broke, Lily dialed the number for Blue Taxi Cab Company.

"Hello. I'm trying to locate one of your drivers who works at night. Her name is Pearl. I need to speak with her right away. Today. Yes, today. What? No. Sorry, I don't know her last name. I can describe her for you. Well then, let me speak with your supervisor!" Lily snapped.

"As old women are grateful for death,
Without knowing why;
But feeling a release from the too bright sun,
The too warm days, the too wide sky,
And quick life everywhere,
And being glad they can withdraw again
Into themselves."
— Marion Thompson van Steenwy

CHAPTER 9

Pearl

Pearl Truman sat on the edge of her bed, took off her shoes and wiggled her toes. She stretched her legs out in front of her and sighed. Each time she moved, the bracelets on her arms made a jingling sound, which made her smile. She glanced up at the wall above her bed to the painting of Jesus, then dropped her gaze to the photo of her son on the bedside table. Her smile faded quickly.

Henry. Her dear son Henry. How she would miss that boy forever. If only the law could have caught and fried the devil who murdered him all those years ago in that drive-by shooting, just days before his seventeenth birthday. But that would not have brought her son back. He was gone. Pearl would always be alone now. Her heart felt unbearably heavy in her chest. Maybe her blood pressure was up again.

Well, this was no way to start the first vacation she'd had in five years. Lord, no. She needed to do something fun. Go somewhere. Maybe go to Graceland. She had always loved that Elvis Presley. Why not? Or what about New Orleans? This appealed to her even more. She could go to one of those travel agencies and get some information. In fact, she figured, why not today?

Anticipating this, she ignored the phone when it first rang. Even listened to it ring several times before picking up the receiver.

"Halloo?" she said in her best singsong voice.

"Hey Miss Pearl, it's Emma. You know, from work," the voice said. It was her boss. Pearl cringed a little, wondering if she'd done something wrong.

"Oh hey, Emma," Pearl said, "anything wrong?"

"No, no everything's just fine. And I do apologize for disturbing you on your first day of vacation and all, but the thing of it is, there's this woman who keeps callin' for you. I mean to say, she just will not give up. Seems nice enough. Says her name is Lily Storm and her mama is Annabelle Storm. She told me her mama has that old timer's disease. Says you were real kind to them a number of weeks back. I'm guessin' she just wants to thank you and all. She left her number. You want it?" Emma said, then chuckling added, "Maybe she wants to give you a big tip or something. You know."

"Storm? Oh, why yes, yes ma'am, I do remember that lady," Pearl said, picturing Annabelle in her tennis shoes, nightgown and flowered bathrobe. Pictured her pounding on the door of her Aunt Myrtle's house determined to visit her old auntie in the middle of the night. She surely did have some kind of old timer's disease. "Sure, I'll take the number. I'll call the lady."

She jotted down the number, then made a mental note to call the lady after she returned from the travel agency. She'd made up her mind. It was time for a real vacation.

Hours later, Pearl returned from the travel agency loaded down with maps, tourist guidebooks and motel reservations. She would drive, of course. Hated planes. She had three weeks of time off ahead of her and five years of vacation money saved. She decided she'd take the scenic route. She'd pack light but bring an extra suitcase for all her purchases. Pearl could hear that New Orleans jazz music now. She closed her eyes and hummed an old Louis Armstrong number, her voice getting louder and louder.

Even as she opened her closet to grab a suitcase from the top shelf, something tugged at her. Miss Storm. Oh lordy, I do need to call that sister lady back, she mumbled under her breath. It would only take a minute. She dialed the number.

"Miss Storm, this is Pearl Truman. You know, the taxi cab driver? I had a message you called," Pearl said into the phone. She couldn't tell if it was the mother or daughter who answered.

"Oh, thank God, you've called back. I've been trying to reach you for weeks," the voice said, sounding younger the more she spoke. "Do you remember my mother? She was very confused and had you drive her all the way to Georgetown to visit her aunt who had passed away many years ago?"

"Well, I surely do. I hope ya'll are okay. Can I help you in some way?" Pearl thought about what her boss had said about a big tip. She didn't think that was the reason for the call. Even though she could use the money, she hoped that wasn't it. Too awkward.

"I sure hope so. Do you remember when you took me aside and told me that you had been a caregiver for an elderly woman until she died?" the daughter asked.

"Yes, yes I did indeed say that," Pearl said, hesitant. Where was this leading?

"Pearl, I realize this is totally out of the blue, but is there any way you would consider caring for my mother? She has Alzheimer's disease."

"Oh golly. I don't think I can do that, doll. I'm starting a three week vacation today," Pearl said, then suddenly puzzled, added, "there are all sorts of agencies you can check with. All sorts of folks who do that kind of work—what was your name again, doll?"

"Lily. It's Lily," the daughter said, becoming eerily quiet.

"Now Miss Storm, why would you want me?" Pearl asked. "I've only met you the one time. Why, you don't even know me."

"I know. Crazy, huh? Seems crazy. But Pearl, my mother took a true liking to you. She has run off most everyone I've interviewed. No one has taken the job for more than a few days at a time. She just doesn't like strangers in her house. All she needs is someone to watch her while I'm at work," Lily said, her tone becoming more frantic. "I'm sorry to admit but, I'm desperate."

"You afraid she might run up a big cab fare?" Pearl said.

"Well, yes that. And other things. She's so confused," Lily said. "She just needs someone to sit with her during the day. She's not sick or anything. Just sort of mentally repetitious, you know. Confused. Sometimes really confused. Sometimes she can be a little mean. Well, okay—really mean. But she liked you so well. She doesn't like just anyone."

"Hmmm. Well Miss Lily, I don't know what to say exactly," Pearl said. "Tell you what. Why don't I come by for a little visit? We can talk about this."

"How soon can you be here?"

Lily gave Pearl brief directions. But Pearl Truman was as familiar with the city as she was with the act of breathing. She had one of those photographic memories when it came to city streets. It would take her about twenty minutes to get to the west side of the city what with the morning traffic. She would never have suggested coming by to visit, but the daughter seemed so distressed. Pearl felt sorry for her. For the both of them. It might help just to stop by to visit them. Might help the daughter put things in proper perspective. That daughter surely wasn't thinking straight. Lord in heaven, who would go and hire someone they'd only met one time? What kind of sense did that make? Besides, Pearl was about to go on her vacation. To New Orleans. To hear some live jazz music.

The Storm's house looked different in the daylight. It seemed larger, the yard more manicured. The house was colorless and somehow hermetically sealed off from the world. With the exception of two flower gardens spilling over with yellow lantana, blue plumbago and mounds of pink skullcap on either side of the front walkway, the house had a bleak, uninviting look to it. A silent, no trespassing feeling. Pearl felt as though she faded into the scenery in her khaki pants, beige blouse and tan sandals. She'd lost her flair for fashionable colors after Henry's death.

The front door opened before Pearl had a chance to knock. Lily Storm welcomed her in immediately. Pearl couldn't help think how odd it seemed that she would be called to this home where this unfortunate mother and daughter continued to struggle through their days together. She was overwhelmed with sadness for them but also perplexed by the daughter's seeming lack of caution. How could Lily Storm know that Pearl had even been telling the truth about having cared for an elderly woman? Perhaps Lily truly was, just that desperate. Well, no matter, Pearl thought, I just came by for a quick visit. Maybe give the daughter some tips on how to find the right person to care for her mother.

"You got here very quickly," Lily was saying. "Can I offer you anything? Some iced tea? Water?" She led Pearl through the darkened foyer into a large living room with high ceilings and sky lights.

"How nice, but no thank you. I'm fine. Where's your mama?" Pearl adjusted her eyes to the dim interior light. The house was cool, spacious and dark. Nothing like her little two bedroom, one and a half bath, linoleum floor house with its open windows, solid porches and century old live oaks to shade it all year long.

"Mother? Mother, look who's here," Lily said, turning away from Pearl. "It's Pearl. Remember? Your cab driver."

There was no answer. Pearl watched as Annabelle Storm walked into the room. It was sister lady all right, but she looked wretched. She was pale, thin, and the expression on her face was a total blank. Pearl saw that her eyes looked sunken, she had bruises on her arms and a sling partially covering a cast on her left forearm. This was not the same confident, regal, albeit befuddled lady she had driven all over town several weeks ago.

"Mother, you remember Pearl, don't you?" Lily asked again.

"Pearl," Annabelle finally repeated the name. She took tentative steps toward Pearl and stopped. She tipped her head, then smiled. A large welcoming smile, but not one of recognition. "Wonderful to see you. No, we have not met before."

"Hello, sister lady, good to see you. Now let me see. I surely do remember you, but of course, you might'nt remember me all that well by now," Pearl said. Then extending her hand, she added, "Wonderful to see you. You okay today?"

"Uh-huh. I am fine, thank you," Annabelle said, now beaming, eyes shining, but not understanding Pearl's outstretched hand was to shake, and so patted it instead. She was studying Pearl in great detail, the braid extensions, the jangling bracelets, the wide toothed grin. Her eyes began to sparkle, almost dance. She seemed pleased.

"Here, sit and talk, won't you," Annabelle said, tapping the seat of the chair next to the one she sat in, "or do you need to get back to school soon?"

Pearl and Lily exchanged glances. Pearl noticed that Lily, too, looked haggard as though she hadn't slept in a month. She was so determined to keep her mama at home that it was making them both sick, Pearl decided.

"No ma'am, I'm all done with school," Pearl said, turning back to Annabelle who had become preoccupied with a piece of string she'd found on the floor.

"How nice," Annabelle said. "This is my daughter Lily. She's still in school. Lily, would you please bring my guest something to drink. She's quite parched from her travels, and she'll have to go back to school soon. Please, Lily," she waited for Lily to leave, then whispered, "I've been trying to get her to take me home, but she won't do it. Very strong willed, my daughter."

"Kinda like her mama?" Pearl watched as Annabelle tossed back her head and laughed heartily as though this joke was immensely funny. Pearl laughed with her.

Annabelle stood up and with some difficulty moved her chair closer to Pearl.

"Can I go with you?" Annabelle pleaded.

"Go with me? To where? Now, sister lady, where do you think I'm going that would be better than right here?" Pearl said.

"Well, I can't stay here. I won't. My husband is looking for me." Annabelle almost pouted.

Lily returned with three glasses of ice tea, the first of which she gave to Annabelle who did not drink. Pearl took a sip of her tea and almost spit. It was the weakest, most vile beverage she'd ever tasted. Not that she was much for tea to begin with, but this was akin to vinegar. Pearl set her glass down and cleared her throat.

"You must stay for supper, won't you?" Annabelle still did not touch her glass of tea. Pearl figured Annabelle must have meant lunch since it was only ten o'clock in the morning. She wondered if Lily was better at cooking than making iced tea.

"Oh my god, this is terrible," Lily said suddenly as she took a drink from the tea," it's awful, I'm so sorry. I'm not much for making tea, I guess. Actually, I'm sort of a lousy cook, too. My ex-fiancé was a fabulous cook. Chef, actually. He's a chef. We were together for many, many years. I forgot how to cook anything. But you are welcome to stay for lunch. If you don't mind canned soup."

"No, no don't you worry none about me," Pearl considered marching into the kitchen and making a proper pitcher of iced tea. Maybe scrounge up something better than canned soup for these women. No wonder they were both so scrawny. "So, you never married the chef?"

"No, no, it became, uh, too complicated," Lily answered, casting a sidelong glance at Annabelle. "Mother never liked him. She thought he was all wrong for me. I guess he got tired of trying to prove himself year after year. Just finally gave up one day."

There was a biting bitterness in Lily's tone. The mother and daughter locked eyes for a moment. A silent challenge, until Annabelle looked away, her expression becoming vacant. Had Annabelle truly been responsible for the break-up, Pearl wondered. There was a palpable tension between the two women that had been evident from the first time Pearl had met them.

Annabelle stood up suddenly, brushing invisible lint from her jeans. Without a word, she picked up her untouched ice tea from the table and walked toward the kitchen as though someone was calling her. Pearl and Lily watched her leave in silence. Lily moved to the edge of her chair, craning her neck to peer into the kitchen. She glanced at Pearl and smiled a troubled, preoccupied smile.

This is how she lives now, thought Pearl, always worrying about what her mama might be doing next. She did need someone she could trust. But she needed someone with references and maybe even a nursing assistant certificate. Someone who knew basic first aid, basic medical skills. And yet, that would likely be too clinical for Lily.

Pearl figured Lily was really looking for a companion for her mama. Someone her mama liked and would trust. This was the only way Lily would be able to leave her, even for short periods of time. She was either extremely devoted to Annabelle, or else there was some underlying guilt there. Something not yet resolved. Or perhaps she was afraid of her mama. Maybe Annabelle still had some sort of hold on her.

"You're gonna need someone for a long time, Lily. My vacation is for only three weeks," Pearl said.

Suddenly there was a crashing sound of breaking glass, a thud and Annabelle's voice from the kitchen calling out, "In here, glass—oh no…"

Pearl and Lily sprang to their feet in unison and ran to the kitchen where they found Annabelle sitting on the floor next to what appeared to be her shattered iced tea glass and dozens of boxes of Girl Scout cookies. Her back was against a chair, which she had evidently moved to stand on to retrieve the cookies from the top shelf of the cupboard. She seemed dazed, even frightened. Her hair was loosened from its braid and now fell carelessly to one side of her face. There were beads of sweat on her upper lip. Her white blouse was splashed with tea. Broken glass was on either side of her. Something about her mouth didn't seem right to Pearl.

"You hurt, sister lady?" Pearl said, hunkering down to Annabelle's level. "What happened?"

"Mother, are you okay? Did you hurt yourself?" Lily demanded as she glanced around the room. "What were you trying to do in here? Why are all these cookie boxes on—"

"Shh—shh! Hush, now. Something ain't right here," Pearl said, waving her hand in Lily's direction to silence her. Annabelle looked too pale. Her mouth was slack on one side and her eyes were too distant, unseeing. "You hearing me, sister lady?"

"Mmmhmm," Annabelle mumbled. Her voice was weak, almost too soft to hear.

"Who am I?" Pearl asked.

"Shis lobol."

"Who are you?" Pearl asked, getting closer to Annabelle's face.

"Shi ladel."

Pearl turned to Lily. "She either hit her head or is having a stroke. Call 911," she ordered. She watched cold panic shoot across Lily's face as she moved towards the phone. "It's gonna be okay. Just make the call. Tell them to hurry."

Pearl sat heavily on the floor next to Annabelle. She took Annabelle's hand and began to sing her softest version of "When the Saint's Come Marching In." Annabelle's eyes seemed to come into focus. Pearl continued the song.

When the paramedics arrived, Pearl took Lily aside and told her in the only way she knew how that Lily needed to get familiar with reality and send her mama to a home where she could be safe and cared for properly. She also told her that whatever it was that was wrong between the two of them, that trying to care for her at home was surely not the way to make things right.

When she drove away later, Pearl knew in her heart why she'd been sent to the Storm's house once again, thanked God for it, then began planning her trip to New Orleans.

"She's just north
Of the border
Of insanity
Where she's been digging
A little grave
For reality"
— L. Storm

Chapter 10

Clancy

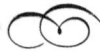

Rain clouds loomed on the horizon, taunting the midday sun. Even the blue of wide open sky seemed scorching, unrelenting. It was the end of another Texas July. A time of drought and soaring temperatures. A time of wilting humidity, the air too heavy to breathe, a residue of dampness coating every living thing.

Ernest Finley stood under the shade of a live oak in the courtyard of the Rainy Alzheimer's Center, shading his eyes against the heat of day. He mopped his forehead with a soggy tissue, then looked in the direction of the rain clouds. Clancy watched him inattentively from the nurse's lounge window.

At that moment she was thinking of her neighbor, Mr. Eliot, and his little dog Kansas. The dog was hers now. Mr. Eliot had passed away a week before, the day after she'd brought the dog to visit him at the facility where he lived. They had been his only visitors. No surprise his cruel son never came to see him. She remembered Mr. Eliot's tears when he saw Kansas. The dog had nestled under the old man's arm and lay quietly, listening to Mr. Eliot's ragged breathing, his eyes never leaving his owner's face. The dog had loved him unconditionally. He seemed to understand more than a little dog should. It had been their final good-bye.

She shifted her focus back to Ernest Finley, noticing how straight the man's posture was. He had the posture of a young man. It was when he took his slow, deliberate steps that his age was more evident. He seemed content enough. Ate well. Slept soundly. Unremarkable medical problems. Made few attempts to escape the locked doors. He never became combative, never uncooperative with staff. His level of cognition was unchanged. He was able to speak. In fact, he spoke with near clarity at times. It was just that he wouldn't. He just would not speak. Rarely had anyone been able to get him to talk. In all the time Clancy had known him, he'd only had the one visitor. The movie star woman who had never returned.

Clancy sighed. She smoothed her long hair and swept it into a ponytail at the base of her neck. After three days off, she was preparing to hear the report from the day nurse. When Mr. Eliot's condition became worse, she'd switched her work hours temporarily to the evening shift so that she could visit him during the day without the risk of running into his wretched son. It would not have been a problem since the son never came anyway. She had been able to work on her sculptures during the day time when she could use the sun as her source of light.

"Hey Clancy, sorry to be so late. You're working alone, again?" the day nurse asked as she entered the nurse's lounge, chart under her arm, stethoscope dangling from her neck. "When're you coming back to day shift?"

The day nurse was a tall, slender woman from Gambia named Mariama. She was the only nurse Clancy found tolerable since working at the Alzheimer's Center. The residents appreciated Mariama's quiet, respectful manner. Despite her impeccable English, they found her accent difficult to understand. Most would simply smile and nod as though it was the dementia causing them to be unable to comprehend her words.

"Hey Mariama," Clancy said, "Yeah, I don't know when I'm coming back exactly. Anything new around here? I've been off for three whole days."

The two nurses exchanged greetings easily, briefly. They sat at the break room table and began the report. Mariama was specific and thorough, giving Clancy full detailed accounts of everything that had happened over the last three days. She reported that Doris Parker was on an antibiotic for a urinary tract infection. Ernest Finley hadn't eaten well for two days, had been seen by the doctor, seemed better now. May Hope's blood thinner dose had been changed.

Mariama continued without pausing. There had been an admission yesterday, she told Clancy. A younger woman, age fifty-two, named Annabelle Storm. She had been admitted from the hospital. Early onset Alzheimer's —probably diagnosed several years ago. She'd had multiple falls and a recent light stroke but had recovered well. Mrs. Storm had multiple medical problems. Mariama listed them in detail. She told Clancy that the woman was very confused. Had not been taking her medicine at home. Had episodes of incontinence. Wandering. Was likely to try to leave but otherwise, a nice lady, cooperative with staff. Quiet for the most part. Sort of an elegant woman, Mariama had added pensively, glancing across the table at Clancy who was writing down everything she was told.

"Elegant?" Clancy repeated as if she were unable to comprehend the nonmedical word. Then looking over the rim of her reading glasses, asked, "Any family?"

"Yes. A daughter," Mariama said. "No other family at all. Her husband was killed in a car accident a few months ago. Mrs. Storm is a good roommate choice for Doris. Doris likes her, I believe."

After Mariama left, Clancy went to find the new resident, Annabelle Storm. She stopped first in the courtyard to check on Ernest, thinking it might be too hot outside for him, knowing how easily heatstroke could take hold of an elderly person. But as she stepped into the courtyard, she saw that Ernest Finley was no longer there. He was no longer standing under the live oak watching the rain clouds roll in off the horizon. Clancy shut the door behind her, returning to the coolness of air conditioning. Too cold for old people, she thought briefly. She passed by Doris Parker who began to follow her but then became distracted by something unseen.

When Clancy finally found Ernest, he was sitting in a chair beside Annabelle Storm who stood staring out the window of her room. Neither of them spoke. The light coming from the window cast a golden hue across the room catching them in its path. They were so still, so quiet. They could have been trapped in an Edward Hopper painting.

"Mrs. Storm?" Clancy said, her voice quiet, trying not to invade the stillness. She watched as Annabelle turned to look at her and was struck by the woman's obvious grace. Like an aging ballerina, Clancy thought. And Mariama was right. Annabelle Storm did have a sort of wise elegance to her. The usual vacant expression of Alzheimer's disease clashed with a look of unresolved pain, something haunting her even as she lost her sense of self. Her face was etched with fine lines of apprehension. "My name is Clancy, I'm one of your nurses."

"Nurse?" Annabelle raised her eyebrows slightly. "Oh, well goodness, thank you, but I don't need a nurse. I'm waiting for my daughter to pick me up."

Clancy saw that her new resident was pale, had diffuse bruising, especially on her arms, eyes mildly sunken, skin turgor poor, and frail, poorly nourished. She was alert enough, confused obviously. Speech clear. Able to ambulate unassisted. She was clean, neat. Her overall demeanor appeared to be calm, not agitated. She clearly didn't mind the presence of Ernest Finley. And Ernest seemed completely content sitting in the soft overstuffed chair that belonged to Annabelle's roommate Doris. There was a framed photo on Annabelle's bedside table of a stately, unsmiling man with graying hair and chiseled features. Clancy assumed it was Annabelle's husband. Her daughter must have placed it there when Annabelle was admitted. For a fleeting moment, Clancy thought it was odd that the daughter had not left a photo of herself.

"Is this your husband?" Clancy picked up the photo.

"Mmm hmm." Annabelle took the photo from Clancy. She held it close to her chest and looked away.

A sudden rush of air stirred behind Clancy, catching her attention. It was Doris entering the room, followed closely by her son. Doris smiled her crooked smile at Clancy, then nodded as if they shared a secret. Clancy looked from Doris to her son and greeted the two as they strolled into the room.

"New roommate, eh?" Doris's son glanced at Annabelle. "Hello, I'm Nate Parker, Doris's son." He extended his hand for Annabelle to take, which she did. She held his hand for a long time, her expression bewildered.

"There are too many people in my house. Let's go on." Annabelle finally dropped Nate's hand. She took Ernest by the arm. He followed her dutifully out of the room.

Just as they stepped into the hallway, a woman began screaming. Screaming so loud that everyone around her stopped to stare. Annabelle and Ernest walked quickly in the other direction. The resident screamer was a wiry little woman named Gloria Perez whose screams were piercing enough to shatter glass. Clancy cringed, excused herself from Doris and Nate to check on the woman. She was met by Carlos in the hallway who was attempting to calm Gloria.

"What's wrong *Señora* Perez? *Qué paso?*" Carlos was shouting, trying to be heard over the screaming.

"Well, you stupid little dip, didn't you see her try to hit my bicycle?" Gloria snapped at him, her dark eyes flashing. She stood halfway up out of her wheelchair to lunge at May Hope, who desperately attempted to wheel past her. The wheels of the two chairs had somehow become locked together.

"I did not, didn't, didn't. Liar, you're a liar. Flyer, dinky smart. Feeney scob. Mutsgug barb! Hell its its! Help! Help me! Help me, help me, help me, hep me! Hep! Hep!" May screeched, still trying to move forward. Her face was crimson red, her eyes filling with angry tears.

"I saw it! I saw what happened! I saw what happened," a resident yelled from the other end of the hall.

"Shut up! Just shut up!" another woman shouted coming up behind the locked wheelchairs. "Why can't you shut up? I'm going to call the police if you don't stop!"

Gloria Perez threw back her head and turned her scream into a full yodel just as Carlos unhooked the two wheelchairs, "Yo, yo, yo, yo, yodalee-oh-lee-oh-lee-oh!"

The screaming, yodeling and cursing had reached a frenzied pitch. Clancy began quickly moving residents away from each other to quiet areas, while Carlos wheeled Gloria out to the courtyard. As they did this, Clancy glanced over her shoulder and saw that Annabelle and Ernest were sitting together on the dayroom sofa, their eyes glued to the wide screen television. An old black and white movie was playing. Their view of the television was partially blocked by a female resident standing six inches from the screen, her open hand resting on Humphrey Bogart's face.

It was later during lunch that Clancy noticed Annabelle and Ernest were still together. They sat quietly at the lunch table, side by side, slightly detached, and yet openly aware of each other's presence. Ernest had given Annabelle most of the food from his tray. She ate very little. Said even less.

When the nursing assistant tried to coax the two into eating their meals, Annabelle told her that she'd already eaten. Ernest mimicked what Annabelle had said, telling the assistant that he had already eaten as well. There was something about the two that seemed connected. Maybe it was their temperaments, or perhaps they each were reminded of someone from the past when they looked at each other. It happened sometimes, Clancy thought. Sometimes people with Alzheimer's just gravitate toward each other, defying any sort of rational explanation.

Clancy believed in her heart that it would be a blessing for Dr. Finley to be able to share his days with someone. He had been so alone. His time was spent standing in the courtyard on fair weather days and inside staring out on days of rain. He never had interacted with anyone that she had seen. He was pleasant with the staff, but if anyone attempted to engage him in conversation, he would simply smile and walk away. Every once in a while, he would try the locked door again, giving it a half-hearted tug, then stare through the glass into the long hallway that led to the administrative offices. If someone came through the doors, he would politely step back.

In his chart, Clancy had read that Ernest Finley had been an internal medicine doctor. She wondered if any of his former patients knew of his illness. She wondered why no one, absolutely no one except for the movie star woman, had visited him. But then, she decided that he was so private that perhaps no one who had cared about him even knew of his illness. It would make sense that a man like Ernest Finley would tell no one.

Two weeks passed before Annabelle Storm's daughter came to visit her mother. Clancy began to wonder if the daughter had just dumped Annabelle at the facility and then gone on with her own life, glad to be rid of the burden. The thought of it annoyed her. To Clancy, the daughter's absence was an indication of indifference. And to her, indifference translated into neglect. How could this daughter be apathetic about her own mother who Clancy saw as a noble woman trapped in a losing battle of chasing memory shadows? So what if she asked repetitive questions? So what if she couldn't remember how to dress herself correctly? She still deserved a visit from her only living relative, didn't she?

Most days Annabelle was quiet, almost studious. When she became frustrated by her confusion, she would retreat to her room, or any nearby vacant room. She would curl up on someone else's bed and stare at the wall, whispering to herself. Her whispers became frantic at times. There was something about her, some unresolved conflict, some inner turmoil that caused her whole demeanor to exude urgency and unrest. Every evening, she paced the unit's hallways well into the night. Sometimes Ernest Finley would pace with her.

When Annabelle's daughter appeared at the nurse's station for the first time demanding that the man in her mother's room be removed, Clancy knew who she was immediately. She had the same high cheekbones, deep dark eyes and graceful movements as her mother. With the exception of a few chaotic locks, her long hair, not yet gray, was pulled away from her face exactly like Annabelle's. She even wore similar clothes, faded blue jeans and a white knit shirt. Except that, unlike Annabelle's sporty tennis shoes, the daughter wore expensive-looking sandals. Her overall manner was different from Annabelle's though. She was direct and unyielding. It was as though her life had been filled with a multitude of times she'd had to defend herself and now she had no patience for it. Clancy knew her type. She immediately disliked her.

"Don't you have any way of restricting who goes into my mother's room?" Lily asked. Her voice was edgy, confrontational. She glared openly at Clancy. It was evident that she'd already made up her mind that the Rainy Alzheimer's Center was a place filled with flaws and that she would need to be on guard for even the slightest discrepancy. "My mother is Annabelle Storm, room twelve. I'm Lily Storm, her daughter," she added in afterthought, glancing toward her mother's room.

"Oh yes, okay. Annabelle Storm. You want to know if we can restrict who goes in her room? Well, we can to an extent of course, but this is an Alzheimer's unit. People wander." Clancy suddenly felt a flash of defensiveness. "It's what they do. It's why they're here. Some of them. Most, really."

"So, what do you intend to do— in this case? I don't want him there. It's—it's weird," Lily said forcefully, then softening her tone she added, "My father died only a few months ago. She misses him. She doesn't need some strange man hovering around her."

"I'm sorry about your dad. But the thing is, Dr. Finley is a very gentle man. Very quiet. Your mother seems to like the company. It keeps her calm, settled." Clancy felt more and more irritated. What did the daughter think was going to happen anyway? Could she not think past herself long enough to see that her mother was content having him around? "I'm sure it's totally innocent. It's just, you know, companionship."

"Doctor Finley? He's a doctor?" Lily was thrown off guard.

"Well, he's retired. But yeah, Dr. Finley is a—" Clancy started.

"Okay, look, I don't really care about that," Lily interrupted. "Who's in charge here anyway? Are you the nurse?"

"Yes. I'm in charge. My name's Clancy. Clancy Finch. I've been taking care of your mother since she was admitted two weeks ago," Clancy answered crisply, bracing herself for confrontation. She wanted to say—*and where have you been these past two weeks? Why do you all of a sudden come in here acting all concerned about her?*

Clancy glanced past Lily to see Annabelle and Ernest making their way to the courtyard together. They walked slowly, but deliberately, as if someone was calling to them. There arms were linked together. Clancy looked back at Lily who continued to glare at her, oblivious of Annabelle and Ernest's presence behind her.

"Look, I'll do what I can," Clancy shifted her attention back to Lily, "but I really believe their friendship is harmless. It might even do them some good."

"Do them some good? What? No! No, I need for you to fix this. I don't like it. It's just not—not right. My mother is, well, not herself anymore," Lily's tone changed slightly. Clancy thought she heard a slight tremble to Lily's voice, as though she might be suppressing tears. She watched as Lily turned abruptly from her, glanced around the day room, spotted Annabelle and Ernest and followed them outside into the courtyard. The three of them stood awkwardly for a moment, enveloped by the heat of the day, sucking in the heavy air.

From inside, Clancy watched as Lily began speaking to Ernest. Lily's hands were on her hips, her demeanor was severe, scolding. Clancy saw Ernest take steps back, turn away, shove his hands into his pockets and then stand motionless, gazing up into a nearby oak tree. He seemed embarrassed.

Lily took Annabelle by the arm and led her to a bench on the far side of the courtyard. Even as they walked together, Clancy sensed an emotional distance between the two women. Annabelle glanced back at Ernest and motioned for him to come along, but he didn't see her. He seemed horribly lost. Clancy could see he was talking to himself.

"Clancy, could you check Mr. Dickens? He's kind of lethargic," Carlos said coming up behind her. "He was okay earlier. I think he—"

He was interrupted by the sudden shrill ringing of the nurse's station phone. He answered it, then immediately handed it to Clancy. "It's Dr. Duncan, he needs to talk to you about Doris Parker."

Just as he said this, Gloria Perez began screaming from across the room. "She hit me, she hit me!" There was no one anywhere near her. She strained to stand from her wheelchair but kept dropping back into it, almost tipping it over, which seemed to infuriate her even more.

"Clancy! I can't work like this," one of the nursing assistants yelled as she stomped up to the nurse's station, red faced and sweating. "We're too short staffed. How am I supposed to do all this? Everyone keeps pooping. I mean everyone. And all my residents just want to fight me. The other aides keep disappearing. No one will help me! And it's just so freaking hot in here. I'm telling you right now, I'm about to walk out!"

Directly behind the enraged nursing assistant, May Hope teetered precariously past the nurse's station with a look of glee on her face, having left her requisite wheelchair behind. She swayed unsteadily, lost her balance, regained it, then stopped, momentarily distracted by Gloria Perez's screaming, which had escalated into a full yodel.

Clancy could see that Doris Parker's son was standing a few feet from the nurse's station, waiting to speak with her. He smiled and shook his head as if to indicate that he was in no hurry. Clancy turned toward Carlos.

"How lethargic? Is Mr. Dickens responding to you?" Clancy asked, and then without pause, turned to the nursing assistant and said firmly, "I'll talk with you in a few minutes, but right now you have got to get May so she doesn't fall and figure out what's wrong with Gloria. Help her. I mean right now." Clancy turned her back to the nursing assistant, motioned to Doris's son that she would be with him in a moment, then spoke into the phone while glancing up at Carlos. "Dr. Duncan?" she said.

Carlos mouthed words to her, "not real lethargic, just sort of blah. Maybe it's his blood sugar." He shrugged at Clancy as she jotted down orders from the doctor. She nodded vigorously at Carlos and pointed to a carton of orange juice on the counter. Carlos took it and headed for Mr. Dicken's room.

"I'm on my way," Clancy called after him, then said into the phone, "okay, yes, Dr. Duncan, I'll make sure it gets done. Right away. Yes, yes, I'll call the lab. Thanks, thank you, bye." She had to yell to be heard over the screaming Gloria, who was being wheeled away by the angry nursing assistant.

When she turned to speak with Doris's son, he had gone. She felt unexpected disappointment as she rushed after Carlos to Mr. Dicken's room, glancing one last time into the courtyard at Ernest, who now sat looking dejected beside the stone birdbath, gazing into the murky water. On the other side of the courtyard, Annabelle and Lily sat in the deep shade of the live oaks and appeared to be in the throes of an argument. Annabelle was fanning herself with a folded newspaper. The earlier tier of rain clouds had dissipated, leaving a blazing summer sun to dominate the sky, wilting everything in its path except for a lone Mexican firebush.

During the weeks that followed, Lily came every evening to visit her mother. She must have sensed Clancy's dislike for her, because she always breezed past the nurse's station without a greeting. Her pattern became predictable. She would immediately wave Ernest away, then walk her mother out to the courtyard or to her room so that the two of them could visit.

When Annabelle and Lily went to the courtyard, they would sit next to what had once been a vigorous flower garden attended by a former resident. The resident had died a few years back and very few of the flowers had survived the neglect of her absence. Usually Lily would water what was left of the flowers, using a courtyard hose that hadn't been touched in years. Then she would settle next to Annabelle and read from a journal.

A few times Clancy was close enough to hear that Lily was reading poetry and short stories to her mother. Annabelle would fall silent, close her eyes, breathe deeply and listen to the rhythm of the words. Clancy knew Annabelle couldn't have understood the poems, but she seemed to savor them.

Apparently so did Doris Parker's son, Nate. Not long after Lily began visiting her mother on a regular basis, Clancy noticed that Nate and Lily seemed to be having long heartfelt conversations on the days they happened to visit at the same time. To Clancy, they seemed oddly mismatched. The only thing they could possibly have in common was the fact that both their mothers had the same disease.

Following one of Nate's visits with Doris, Clancy discovered a neatly folded note he'd left for Lily on Annabelle's bedside table. Placed on top of the note was a single pink rose. Clancy picked up the rose tentatively, admiring the delicate petals and sweet scent. The stem had no thorns. It was an absolutely perfect rose. She held it to her throat while she unfolded the note. The note turned out to be Nate's slightly awkward invitation to meet with Lily for coffee to talk about poetry, about literature, about their mothers. Since Nate Parker was a literature professor at the university, it seemed logical that he would find Lily Storm interesting for her affinity for poetry. But Lily Storm was nothing like Nate's late wife.

Clancy had never forgotten Nate Parker's wife. At her previous job as a critical care nurse, she'd cared for Mrs. Parker in the final weeks of her terminal illness. The woman had been soft spoken and sweet natured, nothing at all like Lily with her edgy assertiveness. Lily Storm was pretty despite her personality flaws, but Doris's son deserved better. Even if it was just for coffee. Clancy wadded the note into a ball and without even a glance back, dropped it with the pink rose into the hall trash can on her way back to the nurse's station.

"Your mother seems to enjoy the poetry you read to her," Clancy remarked one day weeks later as Lily darted past the nurse's station. She had begrudgingly begun to admire Lily's devotion to her mother. But that was all. She just didn't like the woman's audacity and utter resolve. To her surprise, Lily stopped, turned and smiled at her.

"Yeah, well she doesn't really understand it anymore, but I think she'd always liked reading my short stories and poetry." Lily looked back at her mother who sat with Ernest in the shadows of the dimly lit dining area as though waiting for another meal even though it was past nine o'clock in the evening. Both of them had poor appetites and picked at their food, so their wait for the arrival of a meal seemed oddly displaced.

"It's your poetry? You write poetry?" Clancy followed Lily's gaze toward Annabelle and Ernest.

"Yes. That and short stories. I was an English—well, journalism—major, always have liked to write." Lily tucked a stray lock of hair behind her ear and leaned against the nurse's station. She seemed exhausted. Not so much physically, more of a weary preoccupation, an emotional exhaustion that Clancy had seen far too often in family members.

She had no interest in Lily's academic background. And no interest in knowing anything about Lily, unless it helped her understand Annabelle better. "I've been wondering something about your mother. Something she says really often. Maybe it might make more sense to you."

"What is it?" Lily bristled. She stood up straight, her weariness replaced by a sudden attentiveness.

"Oh well, it's nothing really. It's just that she's asked me several times for her red purse. Or no wait, I think she calls it a pocketbook," Clancy said, adding, "or something like that. Once she said it was a suitcase, I guess. Or maybe a box of some sort."

Lily groaned. She rolled her eyes, her expression became hard. She was no longer the whimsical devoted poet daughter.

"In fact," Clancy continued, "she told me you had it. That I needed to call you and that you would bring it." Clancy knew that Annabelle's obsession with the red purse was likely not based in reality, but still, it seemed to haunt Annabelle. Maybe the daughter knew something about it, but the way Lily's manner had changed so abruptly made Clancy suddenly wary of her.

"I really have no idea what she's talking about," Lily said, the fatigue creeping back into her face. Her shoulders slumped a little. "We drove all the way to our cabin in Minnesota to try and find that stupid red box. Believe me, it's nothing. She'll forget about it soon enough."

As Lily spoke, Annabelle floated out of the shadows to stand behind her. She reached out and softly brushed the back of Lily's arm with her fingertips as though trying to determine who she was. Lily started, then turned almost violently, nearly throwing Annabelle off balance. The two women glared at each other. Clancy sensed an incurable hostility between them. Something that could never be right, no matter how much poetry Lily read to her mother. It was something deep and irreversible. Something that only Lily could fix if it wasn't already too late.

"Mother, you startled me." Lily's severe expression changed slowly to mild curiosity.

"Did I?" Annabelle smiled, then turned to Clancy. "She's my sister. This is my sister." Suddenly she was beaming enthusiastically and began to pat Lily's arm vigorously. "Have you met her? Her name is—" she trailed off, but continued smiling.

"Your sister? Mrs. Storm, don't you mean your daughter? Lily, your daughter," Clancy said gently. She watched Annabelle's face cloud with frustration while Lily stared at her mother as though Annabelle was a magician pulling rabbits out of a hat.

"Oh. Oh goodness, what? No, no. Heavens," Annabelle said. She was embarrassed but still not convinced in the least that this was her daughter. "Her name is Hazel—no, I mean, Hazel. Oh, I have to go. There's my husband over there," she added, motioning toward Ernest who waved back at her from the dark dining area.

"Mother, that's not Dad. That's just a man who lives here," Lily said firmly. "Dad isn't here. Mother, are you listening?"

But in an instant, Annabelle was gone. She'd stepped away from Lily into her world of delicate confusion as though she was a spider entering an intricate cobweb. She did not look back. Clancy and Lily watched her glide into the shadows of the dining area.

"Okay, so what if—I mean, what if there actually is a red box somewhere?" Clancy said, still watching Annabelle. "Maybe there's something in it she needed before she reached a stage where she wouldn't be able to ask for it." Even as she said this, she regretted saying it aloud. It sounded illogical. She knew it. She looked down at her hands as she folded them in front of her on the desk.

Clancy knew she was probably the only one who believed that there was transient substance to what her patients told her. She valued what they still had to say while they were still able to form words. Often they said yes when they meant no, and no when they meant yes. Or blurted out the tiniest bits of wisdom in their most frustrated moments.

"My mother doesn't even have a sister," Lily said. She didn't seem to hear Clancy. "I think being around that man is confusing her. Something really needs to be done about that."

Clancy said nothing. The daughter was being unrealistic, denying the obvious. Dr. Finley had nothing to do with Annabelle's declining cognition. It was the disease. It was taking hold of her like quicksand. Annabelle Storm was sinking all by herself. Lily Storm was powerless to stop it. None of her assertions could change it. She would somehow have to discover this inevitable fact on her own in the months that lay ahead.

And Annabelle did continue to decline, as the scorching last days of August slipped unnoticed into sizzling days of September. She rarely spoke in whole sentences and many of her words were nothing more than nonsensical syllables. Even her legs weakened under her, causing her to spend more and more time in a wheelchair. She lost weight. She became dehydrated easily. She succumbed to various infections. Through it all, Annabelle's air of desperate unease never faded.

Ernest continued to follow her, staying with her for long periods of time without a word between them. The Alzheimer's disease had barely progressed in Ernest. He remained the same, with only subtle changes. He seemed distressed as he watched her become more detached, not caring if he was there or not. Unless he walked away. Then she would frantically begin to look for him, not quite sure who it was she was trying to find. If she came upon Doris first, she would stop looking for Ernest. She and Doris would hold hands like children afraid of becoming lost.

"It's a dead baby," Annabelle whispered one afternoon to Doris who was holding a life-like baby doll that belonged to another resident, "dead baabeeee. Can't you see? It's not—it's not—right. Not right," Her words were precise and full of alarm. The doll's head was only inches from Annabelle's face. It glared at her through heavily-lashed blue eyes, its floppy body nearly obscured by the towels Doris had wrapped around it.

"Not either dead," Doris clutched the doll more closely. Her snow white hair was pulled into a short teenage ponytail that bobbed carelessly on the top of her head. She and Annabelle looked like schoolgirls dressed in similar denim jumpers and white sneakers.

Reaching out and touching the doll tentatively, Annabelle recoiled, shaking her head, "dead baaybee, dead, dead," and began to cry. Doris, too, started to whimper and in her haste to comfort Annabelle, she dropped the doll to the floor with a thud. Both women stopped crying, gasped, then stared at the doll. But suddenly the doll on the floor had no meaning for either of them anymore. When Ernest stooped to retrieve it, the women watched as he plopped the doll into a distorted heap of arms, legs, torso and head onto the table as though it was a rejected centerpiece. He sat like a complacent hero next to Annabelle and Doris just as Gloria Perez rolled her wheelchair up to the table.

"You'd better give that baby to me right now. He's mine, you're not supposed to have my baby," Gloria shouted on the verge of a yodeling spree. She grabbed the doll, glaring at the women, poised for a fight.

From behind the nurse's station, Clancy watched as Annabelle, Ernest and Doris simply stared back at Gloria as if she were an actress on a television show. Annabelle looked away. Ernest yawned. A full minute passed. Doris turned to Annabelle and asked her if she knew how they would be getting home.

Before Annabelle had a chance to answer, Doris sprang to her feet. Her hands flew to her face as she shrieked, "It's my son, my son is here. Look, it's my son. I haven't seen him for so long!"

Clancy had come to expect this reaction from Doris each time her son came to visit, no matter how close together the visits were. Doris's mind held no memory of his visits. He could visit her in the morning, come back the same afternoon and have the same reaction from her. She would grab hold of his hands and smile into his face with tears in her eyes, as though he had just come home from the war. If her behavior embarrassed him in any way, he never showed it. Clancy waved at Nate Parker as he hugged his mother. He nodded at her and smiled, turning to greet Carlos who was wheeling Gloria back to her room.

When Lily Storm arrived thirty minutes later to visit her mother, Clancy noticed the impassive way Annabelle greeted her daughter. The greeting was cordial, gracious, with her usual elegance. It was as if Lily had been there all along. And she obviously recognized Lily. Annabelle knew her daughter. Or perhaps it was just that she knew Lily was someone important to her. Annabelle no longer called Lily by name. And as difficult as this was for Lily to accept, she had no choice. She could not make Annabelle remember.

Lily acknowledged her mother with her usual odd reserve that had made Clancy dislike her from the start. She took Annabelle by the arm and led her to the courtyard with Ernest lagging a few steps behind.

The day was hot, windy, the air dry. Scorched leaves swirled around the courtyard, crackling against heated slabs of walkway. They sat on a swing in the deep shade of the live oaks near Doris and her son Nate. Lily burrowed in between Ernest and Annabelle like a chaperone at a high school dance. The three of them simultaneously rested their heads on the back of the swing and sighed. Lily had given up chasing Ernest away weeks before when Clancy had icily informed her that he had no family of his own. It almost seemed as though Lily's visit was as much for him now as her mother. And for some reason Clancy did not understand, there were times when Ernest would call Lily by her name.

Clancy watched with mild fascination as Nate moved Doris closer to Lily as she began to read poems from her journal. Doris's nonsensical chattering was instantly hushed. She folded her hands in her lap, tipped her head to one side and nodded every so often in approval as she listened to Lily. Clancy had heard how soothing and melodic Lily's voice was when she read, and for a moment she felt ashamed that she'd discarded the rose and note Nate had left on Annabelle's bedside table.

Clancy knew it was true that not all of her patients would have listened quietly while Lily read. Despite Lily's animated expressions and compelling voice inflections, their attention would have strayed within mere minutes. But these three sat with Lily and Nate until nearly dusk, listening to short stories and poetry they couldn't possibly understand, content to let the sound of the words be tossed around them like leaves in the hot winds of the September evening.

"While the sun reclaimed its honor
by grazing
Upon unseen meadows,
through delicate
And mannered apple blossoms,
I slept
With your memory"
— Diane Schonblom

Chapter 11

Annabelle

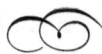

The whisper of hushed voices from somewhere in the darkness jolted Annabelle into a upright position in her chair. She listened closely. The whispering stopped. Had it been her imagination? But there it was again. It must be Lily, she thought. Lily, sneaking in with her friends way past curfew.

Annabelle reached for the lamp switch. She fumbled uselessly in the dark but then suddenly remembered moving the lamp earlier in the day and stopped groping for it. She listened to her own breathing as the darkness became still again. Everything around her had an indistinct shape. It was as though someone had covered her from head to toe in a loosely woven blanket, jammed cotton in her ears and shut off the lights. She could feel the book she'd been reading laying open in her lap, the pages dog-eared and worn.

"Lily, is that you?" she said cautiously, peering into the darkness around her.

Silence. Then laughter. Music. More laughter. Two voices. And then more music, not the kind of music Lily listened to with her friends. It was a bold symphonic piece. The kind of music that accompanied screen-plays.

Annabelle sighed, realizing that she was hearing the downstairs television. And realizing, too, that she must have left it on when she'd come upstairs to read her book. What time could it be? Was it late already? She reached out for the phone and felt relieved to find it cradled in the place she'd left it. She should call Tess's mother. Surely Lily and Tess must have lost track of time. Those girls always did. Especially now that they saw each other only during the summer months. Since the move to Texas ten years before when Lily was six, she and Tess had remained close friends despite the distance.

Annabelle was fond of Tess. Still, there was something about the girl that made her uneasy. The girl was pretty and popular in her school. She seemed to always have an array of boyfriends until she settled on that Sam Olson boy who seemed quite bright and promising. Sometimes the girls would double date if Annabelle and Stanley approved. Lately though, it seemed that the girls were more secretive about their activities. And the more se-cretive they became, the more polite they were to their parents. The politeness seemed exaggerated, phony, like a cover for whatever they were really doing.

The grandfather clock chimed from downstairs. An-nabelle counted each chime, realizing as it finished that it was only ten o'clock. Lily still had an hour before she was expected to return home. Okay, Annabelle thought. Yes, she was probably too strict with her daughter. And yes, Stanley was the more permissive parent. And yes, Lily favored him because of it, but Annabelle had her rea-sons. She didn't want to be influenced by Lily's favorit-ism. She just couldn't be.

Annabelle had wanted Stanley to make this late May trip north to the cabin, but he'd had a summer school class to teach and couldn't join them until later in June.

In the meantime, Lily would just have to adhere to Annabelle's rules, which were always more stringent without Stanley to buffer them.

She stood up from her deep cushioned chair and stretched. The book in her lap dropped softly to the floor. In one continuous movement, she picked it up, brushed it off, then reached for the light switch on the wall. Squinting against the sudden blast of artificial light, she looked down at the book in her hands. Her girlhood diary. Annabelle had been reading an entry she'd written when she was Lily's age. She had been thinking of her own parent's rigidity. Of their narrow way of thinking, their stern approach to anything that didn't fit with their own values. It was no wonder Annabelle had rebelled so dramatically. No wonder at all.

But she had learned. She had learned some difficult lessons along the way. And she took the knowledge with her into adulthood. She spread it into Lily's life. She promised herself that Lily wouldn't follow in her footsteps. And Stanley had supported her in this. Always. He was the only one who truly understood.

She was thinking of Stanley when the phone beside her started ringing.

"Hello? Stanley?"

"No, no, it's Dottie," Tess's mother sounded rushed as usual. Annabelle couldn't imagine how a person could sound so hurried at ten o'clock at night. "Listen, Lily would like to stay over here tonight. It's fine with me. They're having such fun with their friends. They've gone to a party and will be back in about thirty minutes or so."

"Friends? Party? I thought the two of them were going to a movie. Lily told me they were going to a movie," Annabelle despised any change of plans. She felt physically shoved backwards.

"Well, yes," Dottie forced a light laugh, "they'd intended to do just that, but Sam had a friend playing in some band at a party over in Beau Lake and well, I felt that you wouldn't mind since it was Sam. You know Sam is a very responsible boy, Annabelle."

"I know that Dottie," Annabelle snapped, feeling a wave of anger rise in her. "I just wished you'd told me about it before they left. Beau Lake is nearly fifteen miles away."

"Yes, yes, I'm so sorry, but I do know the parents involved. Very decent country people. It's a party, you know. Sam's friends have a band."

"I'll have to call you back," Annabelle slammed the phone into the receiver then abruptly picked it up again and called Stanley.

"Mmm—hello?" Stanley answered on the first ring, sounding half asleep. Annabelle pictured him in his plaid boxers and white T-shirt, sprawled across the bed, the phone propped under his chin, squinting to read the alarm clock, running his hands through his tousled graying hair, reaching for, but missing his glasses that would be neatly tucked into their case on the night stand.

"Stanley," Annabelle blurted, not waiting for an exchange of greetings, "Lily and Tess have gone to Beau Lake to a party with Sam Olson. To Beau Lake, Stanley. You know how I feel about that town. The party is on the property of someone Dottie knows, but she didn't tell me about it until just now. I don't like this. I thought Lily was at the movies with Tess. Stanley, I'm furious. I don't know what to do. What should I do? Should I drive over there and get her?"

"Whoa. Hold on Annabelle," Stanley was fully awake now. "Wait a minute. No, no. Do not go get her. I'm sure it's fine. I don't think Dottie would let Tess and Lily go off just anywhere. She's going to make sure those girls are safe."

"She said that Lily wants to stay at Tess's tonight, too. Stanley? I just don't think—"

"Annabelle, really, it's okay. Let Lily and Tess have some fun. They're sixteen. They're good kids. Tell you what. Call Dottie back and ask her to have Lily call you when she gets in, okay?"

"Well, if you think—" Annabelle agreed to call Dottie back.

"It'll be fine, Annabelle," Stanley said, then added, "Whatever you do, Annabelle, please do not go get Lily, okay?"

"Alright Stanley, I won't."

"Okay, good. Did you get rid of those old letters and diaries yet?" Stanley said, changing the subject.

"No. Stanley, I'm sorry, I didn't," Annabelle apologized, embarrassed.

"Annabelle, we talked about this," Stanley began gently.

"I know, I know. But I just need—I just want to hold on to them for a bit longer. I can't explain it. It's just the memories of—can you try to understand?" Annabelle said. "Such good things came from bad. Sometimes, I have to remember. I want to—remember. I want forgetting to be—to be—a decision. You know, a conscious decision to forget. I don't want to forget things just because they're stolen away from me."

"Annabelle, I do understand. You know that. But you know your memories won't ever be stolen away from you. You won't forget about things from the past." He sighed, "but, I suppose if you insist on holding on to all that stuff, it's okay. For a while. Only for a while though. Like we talked about. It's not a good idea for it to be lying around."

He paused, then added more cheerfully, "Anyway, go look in the boathouse. I built a small pine chest last year. It's on the shelf towards the back. Well, it's really

just a box, but you can put everything in there and lock
it. There's a padlock inside. It can be a box for your
mementos for the time being. When I come up to the
cabin next month, we'll store it away or else we'll bring
it back with us to Texas, okay?"

"Okay."

"Eventually when you decide, we'll destroy it all.
We'll just take the whole thing to the Colorado River
and let it go with the current."

"Or maybe burn it," Annabelle said.

"Or that."

After they hung up, Annabelle walked to the dresser
mirror, picked up her hairbrush and began brushing
her hair. Or what was left of her hair since she'd had
it cut into a short bob. She hated the style. It made her
look like a child with huge eyes, a tiny face and lanky
body. She'd only had her long locks chopped off because
of a comment she'd overheard Lily make to her friends
about how outdated Annabelle's hairstyle was. Especially compared to their mother's hairstyles, Lily had
added. Like Tess's mother. Always wearing the latest
fashions. Always knew what was popular with the kids
and what wasn't.

Annabelle began yanking the brush through her hair
in short choppy movements until it became caught in a
tangle at the base of her neck. She freed the brush, tossed
it onto the dresser, then walked to the phone and dialed
Dottie's number. The phone rang fourteen times before
a hurried-sounding Dottie picked it up, quickly agreed
to have Lily call Annabelle when she returned from the
party, then ended the call abruptly.

Too abruptly, Annabelle thought. But she would wait
for Lily to call while she went to search for Stanley's
small wooden box in the boathouse. She stepped onto
the hallway landing and looked out through the open
upstairs window towards the old boathouse. A full moon

had punched a hole into the deep blue sky, washing everything in its path with a soft indigo light.

The chilly May air caused Annabelle to shiver. From the distance of the cabin, the boathouse, which was nestled into jack pines and blue spruce, looked dark and mystical. Elongated shadows cast by giant coniferous trees loomed over the rooftop, spilling onto the grassy bank, barely kissing the water's edge. Black lake water splashed against the old stone foundation. The moon poured a path of light across the water onto the shore, illuminating three deer that stood together, alert, wary, tails flicking. Maybe they sensed Annabelle's watchful gaze. She waited. When they moved on, she descended the stairs and walked out into the night.

The boathouse had been her refuge when she was young because of its constant state of abandonment. Her family had owned a boat briefly but sold it when Annabelle was a small child. She had loved the smell of decaying pine needles, of the old wood-paneled walls, the mildew smell of things stored away too long. Her parents never ventured close to the water. Had never, to Annabelle's knowledge, even entered the boathouse. Annabelle had loved the lake, the splash of waves, the spray of cool water on her face. It had always made her laugh.

As a young child she had played along the shore unattended. Her mother had been deathly afraid of water, would not go near it. And as the years went by, her father had never ventured too far from his liquor cabinet. Annabelle's laughter at all the small joys around her was met with coldness, inebriated disinterest.

Her parents shared none of her enthusiasm for anything. The boathouse had been Annabelle's place of escape from their erratic wrath and scrutiny. Scrutiny and harshness born out of the drowning death of her older sister who had been a runaway when Annabelle was too young to understand what any of it meant.

She found the small wooden box immediately. Stanley had polished the knotty pine and built a perfect little storage container complete with brass hinges and latch. Inside was a shiny padlock with two keys. She removed the padlock and keys and placed her tattered journal, stack of worn letters and photos at the bottom of the box. She stared at the neatly stacked contents and suddenly gasped. Something was dreadfully wrong. The box looked like a small coffin. Like a memory coffin. She shuddered, then snatched the journal, photos and letters quickly out of the box. She held them to her chest like an infant.

She looked around the boathouse. Several cans of paint and brushes lined a shelf above her. At that moment she knew she would have to paint the box despite the beautiful knotty wood. She would have to. She couldn't lock her letters and journal into a coffin. It was just too eerie. She decided on a can of red paint. Red to signify the tormented ruins of years past, red to obliterate the sarcophagus storing of things close to her heart.

By the time she was finished painting, Annabelle could hear the grandfather clock chime eleven times through the open windows of the cabin. The phone ringer, which had been turned up to high, had not rung. Lily hadn't called. Annabelle started back towards the cabin with the intention of calling Dottie, a combination of dread and rage welling inside her. No, Stanley, I won't go get her, I promise. Stanley was always right about these things, wasn't he?

Just as she got to the back door, Annabelle turned sharply and walked to the car. She would go. No one would see her. She would go to Dottie's and secretly make sure her daughter returned from the party. That's all. No one would ever even know. She would never tell anyone that she'd spied on her sixteen-year-old daughter.

Annabelle peered into the night behind the wheel of the old Ford station wagon as she drove slowly along the lake road, turning onto the more remote back roads to Dottie's house. Even by the light of the full moon, she had trouble seeing ahead of her. No one had ever wanted to ride with her on a drive like this because of her jerky stop-and-start style of driving. Stanley had joked about bringing air sickness bags along. It was true. She was a horrid driver. It was just that she had promised herself that she would never hit a deer or any other animal crossing the road. And, too, she had never been comfortable driving the big station wagon. It was too much car for her. Stanley usually drove them wherever they needed to go. It was understood.

When she reached the outskirts of Dottie's property, Annabelle dimmed the headlights the way she'd seen private investigators do on television. She felt confident, in complete control. No one would see her. She just wanted to see that her daughter made it back safely.

The house was on the outskirts of town, nearly hidden by a stand of young poplar and birch trees swaying in the night breeze. Annabelle parked the car across the road, cut the engine and slumped into a comfortable position in her seat. She could see the front door and most of the driveway.

The house looked nearly uninhabited. A lone amber lamp glowing from the living room and a tiny hint of light coming from the kitchen made it appear that someone inside was waiting for someone else. Annabelle concluded that Lily and Tess must not have returned from the party. The hands of the clock on the dashboard had moved to midnight.

Lily had already broken her curfew by an hour. Annabelle was furious. At Lily. At Dottie. At Tess. At Sam

Olson, his friends and their band. At the parents who let the kids have a party. And then, at her own parents for being so strict, so heavy handed with her and yet somehow not caring about where she was or what she was doing.

Had her own parents ever cared about her at all? Annabelle had a vague recollection of her older sister holding her as a young child, singing to her, whispering to her gently, earnestly. Her sister had made cooing sounds like a dove that had made Annabelle giggle, had made her feel happy, made her feel safe, while the two of them swayed in a giant wooden rocker beside the open window of her room. She remembered the stir of a warm breeze and the feel of lace curtains sweeping softly across her face. She thought she remembered the dampness of her sister's tears as she kissed Annabelle on the nose. And then, suddenly, her sister was gone. The coddling and softness vanished forever.

All that Annabelle would ever know of her sister was what she would learn from listening to her parents speak in hushed voices behind closed doors. When Annabelle was little, she'd pieced enough parts together to know that her older sister had run away, come back, and then there was the drowning that happened on a summer day, heavy with dark clouds of a storm that never came. She knew that her sister's name had been Hazel. And, in time, she discovered that no one would ever speak of her again.

When Annabelle was a young girl, her parents had barely tolerated her cheerful antics. They begrudgingly endured her fun-loving nature. But by the time she was Hazel's age, they'd become obsessed with controlling her, admonishing her for her lack of ambition and poor choices. It was the only time in her life that she'd actually been truly afraid of her parents. Afraid of what they might do or say to her in the name of their irrational religion and their apathy. Terrified that God was on their side. Afraid that if she didn't do as they told her, believe what they said, that she might die young and be hurled headlong into the depths of hell.

Suddenly headlights filled the Ford's rearview mirror as a Mustang convertible screeched into view, then swerved haphazardly into the driveway. Annabelle ducked out of sight, hoping her station wagon wouldn't be recognized. She could hear the loud thud of rock music mixed with the squeal of laughing teenagers. Without even looking, Annabelle figured there were too many kids in the car. Kids coming from a rowdy party. Good kids just having fun and bad kids taking insane risks, influencing all the others. The car turned into the driveway stirring up gravel as the tires screeched in protest. Annabelle sunk deeply into the front seat of her car.

Once the convertible stopped in the driveway, the engine was cut and the music abruptly died. Annabelle peered over the steering wheel and was surprised to see instead a car full of kids there were only four. Lily, Tess, Sam Olson and some other boy. Some other unidentified boy with long unruly hair, leather jacket and torn jeans, who now grabbed Lily's arm and pulled her to him with a swagger that made Annabelle believe he'd been drinking. She shot up in her seat and watched them.

But the wild boy had pulled Lily into the shadows, and Annabelle saw nothing. She could only see Sam Olson walking Tess to the front door. She watched him return to his car, lean on the hood, stare up at the full moon and light a cigarette. A cigarette. Had Lily been smoking, too? Drinking? Were drugs involved?

Annabelle's thoughts began to spin. How could Lily even know this boy? They had only been in Minnesota for a few weeks. She felt sick. Stanley's warning of leaving Lily alone interrupted her thoughts. She waited. Her fury was subdued only by a flood of new apprehension. Lily was only sixteen. The boy looked older, more experienced with a rebelliousness that Annabelle loathed. Her daughter was still a child to her. A smart kid with a bright future that would include a university degree, a brilliant career and then, maybe then, she could meet a decent man like Stanley, get married, settle.

Annabelle slumped back into her seat. She could hear the dashboard clock ticking rhythmically like a tiny heartbeat. How could Lily have let her down like this? Annabelle had been very clear about when she expected Lily to return to the cabin. She'd always been clear about dating and parties. All she'd ever asked was to know who Lily would be with, where she would be going and who the parents were. But most parents didn't share Annabelle's ideas. There were many parties and dates Annabelle had not approved.

Annabelle had half a mind to storm up to Dottie's house and ask her why she had been so dishonest with her. And just why she'd decided that it was preferable to shield Lily from her own mother whose only concern was for her daughter's welfare instead of sending her home at a reasonable hour. Surely, Dottie would call Lily into the house, instruct her to call Annabelle right away. Surely, Dottie would make certain Lily was okay. *She's going to make sure those girls are safe.*

Whatever you do, Annabelle, please do not go and get Lily, okay?

Alright Stanley, I won't.

A reluctant Annabelle turned the key in the ignition, gunning the Ford's engine, not caring if anyone saw or heard her now. She pulled away slowly, straining to see into the shadows. Sam Olson turned to look at her, but then became distracted stomping his cigarette out on the ground. When he turned to look again, the Ford was ten car lengths away, traveling with the stealth of a panther, gravel crunching under the tires.

When Annabelle returned to the cabin, she dropped the car keys on the kitchen counter, then poured herself a glass of red wine. She tipped her head back and swallowed a mouthful of the wine, gagging slightly as the warm liquid shot down her throat. The wine had been set aside for cooking, but Annabelle savored the mildly bitter taste of it anyway. She looked out the window at the moonlit boathouse. A violet cloud was reaching playfully across the face of the stark white moon darkening the land below.

The more Annabelle considered the events of the evening, the more she felt rage boil within her. The rage felt familiar, like a scar that she had picked at until it began to bleed again. Her daughter had defied her instructions. Dottie had ignored her wishes, belittled her concerns. Stanley would not be pleased with any of this. Annabelle knew that. She felt that he would have supported her in punishing Lily for disobeying. There would have to be consequences.

Annabelle climbed the stairs, stopping on the landing to shut the window. The night breeze had turned into a wintry gust of chilled air. Too cool for late spring. She pulled her sweater around her and shivered. She was alone in the house. Every footstep creaked against the old wood floor boards. The cabin had an eeriness to it at night, a screaming silence begging to be unraveled. Annabelle closed her eyes and for the thousandth time sensed her dead sister's presence. Sensed her sister standing firm between Annabelle and the memory of their parents. An involuntary tremor traveled the length of her spine.

Annabelle's daughter didn't know that her room at the cabin had once been occupied by her mother's sister. Lily did not know that her mother had once had a sister. Hazel's room had been empty for all the years Annabelle had lived at home with her parents. The furnishings had been untouched. The old wooden rocker remained by the window overlooking the lake, as though waiting for Hazel to return from the water's depths. Annabelle had been forbidden to enter the room. It was Stanley's idea to let their daughter move into Hazel's room. And Annabelle had agreed, believing that her sister would have been grateful, would have welcomed it.

The floor creaked again as Annabelle stepped into the room and sat delicately on the old rocker, covering her face with her hands. There were so many things Lily would never know. So many things Annabelle wished she could tell her daughter. But it was too late now. Years passed, Lily grew. Time had rolled layers on top of layers of veiled complexities. It seemed impossible to turn back. Annabelle prayed that Lily would follow Stanley's example. That she would embrace the world of academia, become disciplined, make advantageous choices. Yet she was seized by a deep dread that Lily was at a turning point and already becoming a young version of herself. Or even worse, she was becoming like Annabelle's own mother.

As she stood up to leave the room, she noticed Lily's suitcase jutting out from beneath the bed, clothes spilling out onto the floor. She stooped to push it further under the bed, gathering the stray clothes to fold. She was suddenly struck by the skimpiness of the halter top she was holding. And the scanty shorts. And a skirt that caught her attention because it was part of a brightly colored, flashy outfit Annabelle had agreed to let Lily buy the year before when they had taken a trip to London, England. Lily had begged, explaining that the outfit would be more of a souvenir from London than something she would actually wear.

Annabelle arranged the clothes across the bed, then reached to pull the suitcase to her. She began removing more clothes, appalled at what she saw. Where were the clothes she'd approved for Lily to wear? All Annabelle found were tight-fitting tattered jeans, glittery low-cut T-shirts, a black leather vest, spiked heels, even flimsy underwear. These were clothes that screamed of flirting suggestiveness. Clothes that a stripper might wear.

Did Lily not think that Annabelle would see her in these clothes? But no, there were other clothes, clothes hung in the closet that were the outfits Annabelle had purchased for Lily. This suitcase under the bed was filled with clothes that Lily had intended to keep secret from her mother. Clothes that she likely changed into at Tess's house.

Under the clothing, Annabelle discovered an envelope of photos Lily had tucked away into an obscure compartment of the suitcase. Had she been trying to hide it? Annabelle opened it, hesitating momentarily, realizing she was invading her daughter's secret world. But Annabelle believed that secret worlds only led to disaster, to more secrets and more clandestine behavior, driving an irreversible wedge into the mechanism of honorable aspirations.

She took a sharp breath, held it, then exhaled as she began to look through the photos. The photos were of Lily with the reckless long-haired boy she'd seen at Tess's earlier. The two of them were draped over each other, kissing, laughing, gazing into each other's eyes. Who was this boy? Where had Lily met him?

There were other photos of the boy playing guitar in a band. He looked drugged. His hair hung over his eyes, his clothes were beat-up, his whole demeanor exuded danger. Annabelle shuddered, allowing her worry to give rise to anger again. Anger at Lily for being out of her control. Anger that she had a secret boyfriend. Secret clothes. Who knew what else? She might be drinking, doing drugs, having sex. She could get pregnant. Pregnant. Annabelle clenched her fists, her wrath building.

She found scissors in the top drawer of the desk across the room. For a moment she stood beside her sister's old wooden rocker and stared at the array of clothes and photos she'd placed on her daughter's bed. There would be consequences for Lily's actions. Annabelle was certain Stanley would support her in this.

With deliberate certainty, she went to the bed and picked up the skirt from London. She cut it in half. In thirds. In fourths. Into tiny pieces. She watched as brightly colored fabric pieces drifted like loose feathers downward onto the photos of Lily and the unidentified boy. She felt cold, driven by purpose, absorbed by the mechanics of cutting things out of Lily's life.

It became impossible to stop. Annabelle ripped through each photo, separating the boy from her daughter, then cutting him into small pieces. His hair, his eyes, his hands all became nothing. He was gone. A complicated jigsaw puzzle never to be reinstated. She tried to cut through more clothing, but the scissors were too dull. She began ripping, tearing at the clothes, becoming immersed in the task of destroying it all, losing her sense of reason. Her raw anger had been replaced by nothing more than visceral determination.

She didn't hear Lily step into the room behind her. Annabelle turned only as she heard Lily begin to scream. She turned and stood, scissors in hand, gaping at her daughter, not comprehending her presence.

"Mother! What are you doing? Stop! Stop this!" Lily was screaming, then stepping forward cried, "Blood! There's blood all over you! What is wrong with you?"

Annabelle looked down at her sweater, her hands, her fingertips, and saw the color red. Deep red. Streaks and splatters of red. She sucked in a desperate breath, then another and another until her breath began to slow, her head clearing with each breath. It was paint. It was the red paint from the pine box she'd painted earlier that night. There was just enough left on her to look like spattered blood. She almost laughed but stopped herself, regaining her composure, regaining her anger at Lily's behavior.

"It's not blood, it's paint," she said in a smooth voice that surprised even her. "I'm not going to ask for an explanation from you, Lily. I think I have this all figured out. You know what you've done wrong. I want you to clean this up then begin packing. We're leaving tomorrow. This is the end of your summer vacation."

"What? What? That's crazy. It's not even actually summer yet! I can explain—please. Just let me explain, Mother," Lily cried, the indignation in her voice faded into pleading. "Don't you even want to know why I came home early?"

"Oh well, just let me guess. Because you and your friends saw my car at Tess's house? Could that possibly be it?" Annabelle's tone turned surly when she realized that Lily must have changed back into an acceptable outfit before she returned to the cabin. She felt certain that any explanation from Lily now would be a distortion of the truth. She leveled her eyes at her daughter. The lines of Annabelle's face hardened into a mask of resolve. Her mouth was set and determined. There would be no more discussion.

Lily slumped to the floor. She sat in a heap of defeated misery beside the bed where her secret world lay ripped to shreds while Annabelle calmly placed the scissors back in the desk drawer. Annabelle turned, glanced at Lily's bed littered with remains of the suitcase contents, then left the room without a word.

She closed the door behind her daughter's gush of sobs, feeling a sudden surge of unbearable sadness. Slowly, Annabelle sagged to the creaky floorboards, leaning her back against Lily's closed door, running her hands through her short-cropped hair. Hair that had only been cut short so that her daughter might see her as more stylish, more contemporary. More approachable. Annabelle told herself she was a terrible mother. But she felt powerless to stop it.

Things would be better some day. Her daughter would thank her for being so persistent in her efforts to mold her into the best person she could be. Still, sadness welled up in Annabelle like a wave refusing to crash into shore. Sadness that her daughter couldn't be told why she had to be protected from herself. Sadness that her daughter would likely hate her for a long time to come.

"I wait for answers,
Listening
While the candles burn,
And illuminate,
The dancing cherubs
And angelic sculptures
That grace the walls.
They're silent,
And I wait"
— *Diane Schonblom*

CHAPTER 12

Lily

The morning was blistering hot. Hot for so early in the day and too hot for the middle of October. Lily peeled wet strands of hair away from her eyelids with her fingertips, mopping moisture from her forehead with the back of her hand, shielding her face from the sun. The scent of rosemary filled her senses. She surveyed the autumn sky. The ground where she sat digging up irises was warm and damp. Her overalls were smeared with a mixture of dirt and sweat. She glanced over at her mother's old basset hound rolling on the ground, kicking his stubby legs into the air. He'd been fed a belly full of premium dog chow and had been walked around the neighborhood, joyfully marking every mailbox along the way until he had no urine left. Thinking of this, Lily laughed. The dog looked over at her, suddenly at attention, his tail wagging a backbeat thud against the ground.

The next door neighbor stepped out to retrieve his morning paper, spotted Lily and waved. Lily waved back, barely looking up, not wanting to be drawn into a conversation. She had known the Darbys since she was a young girl. She'd attended high school with their son Bob and did occasional pet sitting for their yellow lab also named Bob. Eventually the son went away to a college in the east and became an attorney or stockbroker or something Lily couldn't quite remember. The dog had moved out east with him. Bob and Bob.

"Hello, Lily. How's your mother?" Mr. Darby called to her.

"Oh, well. You know, okay, I guess," Lily called back, watching him cross the lawn towards her.

"We're so sorry, Lily. About your parents. It has to be difficult. First your dad, now your mother. Over such a short period of time. Are you holding up okay?" He looked past her at the house as though it might answer on her behalf.

"Me? I'm fine. You know, good days, bad days. I've decided to sell the house." She followed his gaze toward her parent's home.

"Oh? Yeah, I suppose that makes sense. Annabelle won't be coming back, will she? Such a shame. Such a horrible disease, Alzheimer's," Mr. Darby said as he stroked his chin and shifted his gaze to the endless blue sky. "I remember once when Annabelle came to our front door, trying to find her way back home. It was so strange. We didn't know. You know, about the Alzheimer's."

Lily stood up, sensing Mr. Darby's unease as he talked about Annabelle and Stanley. He'd begun to pace, dabbing his forehead with a handkerchief he'd pulled from his pocket, and sneaking quick glances at her. Did he feel guilty for not doing more to help her parents? She wasn't sure she even wanted to hear what he had to say. It saddened Lily to think of her parents living a secret life filled with distortions and unreality with no one reaching out to help them.

"She finally told us there was a prowler in the house, and she just simply could not go back," Mr. Darby continued. "We'd called the police, only to find out that the prowler was Stanley. She'd locked him in the garage. The doors were all locked from the outside. No telling how long he'd been in there. He looked exhausted. Somehow, he managed to make the whole thing sound like a silly misunderstanding. It was very strange. We decided to forget about it. You know, let it go. There were enough other times when Annabelle seemed just fine."

"Really? I had no idea. Dad never told me any of this," Lily said. She tried to imagine her father locked into the garage for hours, maybe overnight or even days.

"He never told us either. Just left us to wonder. But we sort of knew. We knew something wasn't right." Mr. Darby opened his newspaper without looking at it, then added, "Well, you take care, Lily. Let us know if there's anything we can do."

Lily stared after him after they said good-bye. She watched him disappear into the air-conditioned coolness of his house, wondering what other things he might have noticed about her mother and father during their time of hidden crisis.

Less than a year before, Lily had been in this same spot thinning irises, oblivious to her mother's declining condition. Oblivious that she was taking her father's presence for granted, never once imagining that he could die. Or at least that he could die suddenly. With no good-bye. No preparations. No gradual fading of body and mind. He had been her hero. A dad who could do no wrong. A dad who died too abruptly to be told this.

And now Annabelle was leaving her one degree at a time. There were things Lily still wanted to tell her mother. And even more things she wanted to ask. Lily told herself repeatedly that she was nothing like Annabelle. Never would be. They had nothing in common except Stanley. Had it always been that way? Lily wanted desperately to know where they had gone wrong. There had never been one horrible isolated event, not one specific moment of fury and unforgivable words. They had just always lived in a strained world of deep-seated misunderstanding. For years Lily had blamed Annabelle. Now she blamed herself.

"You are a lucky dog, Caesar." Lily looked back at the dog who stared at her expectantly. And as though the dog might understand her words, she added, "yep, but it's Sunday, we're not going to work today. Instead, big surprise for you old guy, I'm taking you with me to see Annabelle before Tess gets into town."

Lily knew that Tess would be shocked when she saw Annabelle. But she had insisted on coming. She insisted on helping Lily begin the task of sorting through Annabelle and Stanley's belongings. She had convinced Lily to sell her parent's house. Selling the Texas house had been an easy decision. It had always been the Minnesota lake cabin Lily had loved best. That, she would never sell. She loved the legacy, the mystery of it. An underlying mystery her parents had never revealed. Something hushed and sealed away.

Lily sat on the ground next to Caesar and sighed. She was surrounded by unearthed irises. She wiped the back of her hand across her forehead, leaving a streak of dirt just above her eyebrows. The humidity made her feel listless. She looked down at her hands as she picked up the trowel. All of a sudden, she dropped the trowel and stared at her hands. She stretched them in front of her, spreading her fingers, and shuddered. Annabelle's hands. She had never realized that she had her mother's hands. The same square fingernails, the same long tapered fingers, the same pronounced knuckles and veins that made blue rivers just below her skin.

So she had that from Annabelle. That, and their mutual affection for this gnarled old basset hound who now studied her with soulful eyes. The dog had been a gift from Stanley on a day when Annabelle had found a dead sparrow near her bird feeder. She had buried the little bird in the garden and told Stanley how the little birds that came to the feeder were like pets to her, how she had been forbidden to have pets as a child. As she'd said this, her eyes filled with tears. Later that day, Lily's father had returned with a basset puppy. It was one of the rare times Lily saw her mother sparkle with uninhibited animation. And Lily had been immediately jealous of the dog. Jealous of how Annabelle had spoiled him, how he could do no wrong.

It had been her mother's doctor who suggested bringing the dog to visit her at the facility. He'd told her that animals were considered therapeutic for dementia patients. It seemed logical. Dr. Mason had guided Lily through each tentative step of her mother's illness. He'd helped her understand the process of the disease, constantly reminding her that her mother had been diagnosed with early onset Alzheimer's. Reminding her, too, that her father had hidden Annabelle's illness from the world for a long, long time.

Once, Lily had called Dr. Mason in a state of full-blown panic after she had gone to work on Labor Day and found none of her employees there. She had forgotten that it was a holiday and was irritated that they were both so late. She'd called the assistant manager at home but had misdialed and reached a Mexican take-out restaurant listed below his name in her address book. Automatically, she ordered breakfast tacos but then realizing it was a holiday a few minutes later, called the restaurant back to cancel the order.

Annoyed at herself, she drove home. As soon as she reached her front door, she discovered that she'd left her house key at the shop and had to go back. By the time she returned home again, she was seized with the realization that her memory had failed her in rapid succession. She became gripped with a thought that she was experiencing early stages of Alzheimer's. It wasn't until Dr. Mason reassured her that since she had remembered that she'd forgotten, there was nothing to worry about. It took her a day of repeating his words to herself before Lily believed him.

The doctor had been adamant that Lily wait a month before her first visit to the facility after her mother was admitted. He'd told her that Annabelle would adjust more readily if she didn't see her daughter for a while. It made sense, in a way.

When she finally did visit her mother for the first time, the experience was overwhelming. She'd had to enter a special code on a punch pad to enter the place where her mother lived. An elderly woman stood just inside the door with her face pressed to the glass, her eyes filled with frozen desperation. When Lily opened the door, the woman darted past her but was quickly apprehended by two nurse aides who returned her, kicking and screaming, to the dark interior chamber where people wandered aimlessly. For a moment, Lily stood just inside the door, struggling to shake off the feeling that she had just entered a prison, or an insane asylum, or a dungeon. The moment her eyes adjusted to the dim lighting, she spotted her mother across the room.

Annabelle was standing at the far corner of a huge dining area holding a pair of mismatched shoes. Her face was scrubbed clean, her hair brushed back and swept up into girlish ponytail that made Lily think of a doll she'd once had. Her mother wore a red jogging outfit Lily had never seen before. She seemed suspended in space and time, looking straight ahead, smiling. Next to her stood a tall, slender man with piercing blue eyes. Lily thought he looked like Paul Newman. Annabelle and the blue-eyed Paul Newman man were sharing a quiet conversation without making eye contact. Somehow, they seemed attached, and yet detached.

Neither looked at Lily as she approached. Even as Lily called to Annabelle, her mother's expression remained vacant. It had irritated Lily that the man greeted her first. It irritated her more that he wouldn't leave. And that he continued to stand in the space where her father should have stood, as though he belonged. As though there was no where else to go. And when her mother called the man Stanley, Lily took Annabelle by the arm and steered her away from him. She steered her into an overgrown courtyard where they sat together in a creaky, padded swing. Within minutes, Lily discovered that the institutionalized Annabelle was docile, warm, considerate, and nonjudgmental. It seemed too good to be true. She wanted to know this version of her mother.

Lily told the nurse behind the desk that the blue-eyed man was bothering her mother. She told the nurse that his presence was causing Annabelle to be even more confused. The nurse was an attractive, red-haired woman named Clancy who responded with such hostility that Lily had avoided her ever since that first meeting. In time, she could tell that Clancy was an efficient and caring nurse, but her words could abruptly turn sharp and cutting. It was as though she was convinced that her patients had been deserted, and it was her responsibility to inject guilt into the very souls of these family members for this act of abandonment.

Suddenly Caesar began barking. Lily's thoughts were ripped away as she looked from the dog standing at attention to a taxicab pulling into the driveway. She jumped to her feet, dropping iris bulbs to the ground. For a moment she thought it might be Pearl. But it was Tess who flung open the cab door and came toward her with outstretched arms, her blonde hair falling in chaotic curls over her face.

"Tess! I didn't expect you until this afternoon," Lily started, wiping her hands on her overalls. "I was going to pick you up at the airport."

"I know, I know!" Tess gave Lily a quick hug. "I took an earlier flight. I called. You must have not listened to your messages yet. Jeez, you are a mess. Look at you. That dirt streak across your forehead makes you look like you have an alien eyebrow. Actually sort of cool looking. And thin, my gosh. Lily in her element—Lily, the garden nymph."

Together they laughed as Tess paid the cab fare. They took suitcases inside, Caesar trotting in behind them. Suddenly Lily felt safe, carefree. As though she could be a girl again. As though she could say anything that popped into her head. She laughed again, releasing the tension that had burrowed into her bones. If Tess noticed the strain in Lily's demeanor, she didn't mention it. She walked in, gently brushed Lily aside and took over. It was only then that Lily realized that the house was in disarray.

"Okay. You get cleaned up, I'll fix breakfast, we'll eat, then go see Annabelle. Has the dog eaten?" Tess said.

"Of course, he's eaten, I fed him early. Hey, I'm not the one with the Alzheimer's," Lily said, then groaned, "I shouldn't have said that."

The two women fell silent. Tess looked out the kitchen window. Lily folded her arms across her chest and sighed.

"Tess, I'm so sorry, the house is a disaster. I've either been at work or at the nursing home. I'd planned to clean up before you got here." She began wiping the garden dirt from her hands onto her overalls again. She turned, then took exaggerated steps to the shower, stepping out of her garden clogs along the way.

She hadn't realized how hungry she was until she began to eat the eggs and toast Tess had made. She wolfed it down, then licked her fingers while taking a gulp of juice.

"Sorry to be such a pig. I was really hungry. Thanks for making breakfast, Tess,"

Tess nodded, watching Lily eat. There were toast crumbs on her chin.

When they arrived at the Rainy Alzheimer's Center, Tess hesitated, her hand on the door handle. She peered in through the glass, stepped back and turned to Lily.

"I see her," Tess said. "She looks so lost, Lily. Will she know me? Because, you know, Annabelle hasn't always liked me. Are you sure it's a good idea to bring Caesar?"

"Yeah, it's okay. I have permission from the administrative office," Lily said and glanced down at the dog sniffing the floor. "C'mon Tess, it'll be okay. If you feel like you have to leave, its okay. Mother won't know the difference."

"Who is that man beside her?" Tess asked, her hand still gripping the door handle.

"Oh, that's Dr. Finley. Mother's—uh— friend," Lily sighed, aware of Tess's hesitant manner. Ernest Finley was always with Annabelle. It had been only recently that Lily had noticed the inherent loneliness in his eyes. He was quiet. Polite. Blank, in many ways like Annabelle, but kindly, as though it had always been his way.

"Doctor? He's her doctor?" Tess whispered, incredulous. "He's so old."

"What? No, no." Lily started to laugh but stopped herself when she looked back at Ernest, "He's a patient here, Tess. He has Alzheimer's, too. It's just that for some reason he's latched on to Mother. He rarely leaves her side. She seems to enjoy his company. I don't know—I think it's a little creepy," Lily said.

"Oh. Oh, no. I think it's sweet," Tess said.

"You do?"

"Yeah, it's really sweet," Tess said.

"I guess."

"Lily, do you ever think you might get it?"

"Get that it's sweet?"

"No—you know, Alzheimer's," Tess said. "Don't they say that the early onset type runs in families? That it's genetic? I just wondered, I mean, if you ever think about getting—"

"I think about it all the time."

"With forgotten fatigue,
I reach and pass the home
Where I grew up.
There are no children running
Through the backyard,
No dog barking,
No kick the can referee.
Only sounds ricocheting
Through my bloodstream."
— Diane Schonblom

CHAPTER 13

Tess

The moment Tess took Annabelle's hands into hers, she felt a cool sensation of flower petals fluttering to earth. Startled, Tess jerked her hands away, taking a step back. Annabelle smelled of rose-scented talc and stale fruit. She stared at Tess. Her expression was blank. Finally she smiled. It wasn't a smile of recognition, but it was friendly, open, almost childlike.

Tess froze, her mind reeling with memories of a younger Annabelle scolding, humiliating, forbidding Lily to behave like a normal child and teenager. Memories of Annabelle only a few years back, criticizing Lily's career choice, breaking up her engagement. At that moment Tess could only recall the controlling, severe, unaffectionate Annabelle Storm. A person Tess had feared, loathed, puzzled over and sometimes, on rare occasions and for reasons not understood, admired. This woman before her was still regal, still beautiful, still poised, but frail with paper-thin skin and uncomprehending eyes. And vulnerable. So very vulnerable.

Before Tess had time to recover, Lily stepped between them and quickly hugged her mother. The display of affection seemed strained, even forced, but Annabelle didn't pull away as Tess might have expected. A streak of sunlight from the courtyard door illuminated the two women, casting a violet shadow on the wall. The shadow could have been of any mother and daughter greeting each other. Tess looked away.

A painting on the wall behind them caught Tess's attention. It was of a woman wearing an apron over a long dress, her arms folded around a little girl. The child's eyes were shut against the world. Her face was nestled into the woman's apron, her little hands clinging to the woman's skirt. Tess looked from the painting to Lily and Annabelle feeling an immense sadness for the years lost.

"Is he—your doggie?" Annabelle asked suddenly, reaching down to pet Caesar.

"No, Mother. He's your dog. I brought him to see you." Lily glanced at Tess.

"Stanley?" Annabelle's eyes sparkled as she took the dog's face into her hands.

"Stanley? What? No, it's Caesar. Caesar, your dog."

"Oh no, I can't— keep him," Annabelle said with some effort, still petting the dog who sat contentedly at her feet. Her eyes began to fill with tears. Caesar gazed up at her, looking as sad as any basset hound ever could. "I've nothing to feed—him. Nothing. To feed him. I can't take care of—any—anything. Is he your dog?"

"It's okay, Annabelle," Tess said, surprising herself as she hunkered down to the dog's level beside Annabelle, "Lily is taking wonderful care of him."

Annabelle wiped her eyes with the back of her hand and looked up at Tess. She started to speak but only a tiny rush of air escaped her lips. Tess wondered if there had been a quick glimmer of recognition in Annabelle's eyes. But almost instantly it was gone. And Tess thought perhaps she'd only imagined it. She wanted desperately at that moment for Annabelle to remember her, even if the memories were bad ones. She wanted to see her own past come to life in Annabelle's eyes. She wanted to feel an old flash of anger or irritation rise within this woman who had been such a mystery to her.

Suddenly the hush of the dayroom was shattered by a woman's blood-curdling scream from another room. Tess jumped to her feet, "What in the holy hell?"

"It's just Gloria," Lily told her calmly, barely looking up.

Annabelle continued petting her dog.

"Well, she's screaming," Tess snapped. "Don't you hear that? She sounds like she's being killed."

"They're giving her a shower. She always screams like that." Lily sounded weary, almost bored. "Seriously, it happens all the time."

"All the time? How can that be right? I mean, she's screaming like they're killing her," Tess realized her own voice was becoming a shriek. Other residents, family members and staff turned to stare at her. She bit her lip and sank into the chair beside Lily.

"I hate it here," Tess whispered.

"I know. I did at first, too," Lily said. "It's okay though. You'll see. It's not as bad as you might think. Most of the residents are fairly content. You know, peaceful. Well, almost."

"You mean drugged. They're all drugged. They have no idea," Tess rolled her eyes.

"Yeah, well, would that be so bad?" Lily turned to greet a large attractive Hispanic man wearing navy blue scrubs. "Hey, Carlos. How's it going? You look busy."

"Yeah. Kinda am. Looking for a resident." He laughed nervously, his eyes darting around the room. "You okay? Hello Annabelle—"

He was joined by another nursing assistant who also appeared to be searching for someone. They spoke briefly, then split up, walking briskly in opposite directions.

"They lost someone?" Tess asked, disbelieving, her voice raised again, "They actually lost a patient?"

"Resident. They're called residents," Lily said.

"So calling them *patients* isn't politically correct? Well, good lord, how institutionalized sounding is it to call them *residents*? They're still patients in a medical facility, aren't they?" Tess said.

"Over here!" the nursing assistant shouted to Carlos.

Tess watched, incredulous, as Carlos and the other nursing assistant led a short white-haired woman from behind the large screen television. The woman had evidently been there long enough to be considered lost by the staff. She had just been content to stand behind the television, her mind blank with no attempt to find her way out.

"Poor thing, she probably thought she was stuck there," Tess said to Lily. But Lily wasn't watching. Her expression was a mixture of vacancy and boredom. Strands of long brown hair fell over her eyes, but she didn't seem to notice.

Suddenly Tess wanted desperately to leave. How much longer could Lily possibly visit with Annabelle who had nothing to say? Of course there was the dog. And the visit was about bringing the dog. Maybe it would be only a bit longer, Tess thought. But one glance at Lily's complacent manner, Tess knew she had no intention of leaving anytime soon.

"Lily, would you mind terribly if I—" Tess started, then stopped abruptly when Ernest Finley strolled up to them and stood with his hands on the back of Annabelle's chair.

He was wearing a white tank top T-shirt over a pajama top with a red sweater sticking out from under it all. He had tan slacks on underneath his pajama bottoms. Beads of sweat covered his face, and he was having trouble moving his arms. Even worse, he was wearing women's shoes. The shoes were so tight that his feet bulged out over the sides. He nodded at the women as a trickle of sweat dropped into his mouth.

"Lily! Look at him. Oh my god, he's miserable; he's got too many clothes on," Tess whispered, "I mean, for pete's sake, who dressed this poor man? An employee or another resident?"

"He probably dressed himself," Lily said as she smiled up at Ernest. "Tess, it's no big deal, they'll get him dressed properly when they get a chance."

"Get a chance? Are you listening to yourself? Look at him! He's burning up. Someone needs to tend to him right now," Tess raised her voice, which caused Ernest to look away as though ashamed.

"Stanley?" Annabelle turned to him and touched his hand with the tips of her fingers, tapping his knuckles, "this is my husband."

Tess and Lily exchanged quick glances. The expression on Lily's face told Tess to leave it alone.

Ernest said nothing. He just stood staring straight ahead. He reminded Tess of an overstuffed scarecrow in all his layers of clothing, stiff and silent, his mind stolen away.

"Would you like to sit here?" Tess offered, patting the chair next to her. She watched as he dutifully sat beside her. "How are you today, Dr. um—"

"Finley. It's Dr. Finley," Lily said.

Ernest's eyes widened slightly. He tipped his head, but still said nothing.

"He doesn't speak," Lily told Tess.

"Oh," Tess felt suddenly awkward. Maybe words weren't all that important anyway. Maybe he just needed to be called Dr. Finley once in a while. She watched as he bent down to pet Caesar. The dog licked his hand and a huge smile spread across his face.

"He doesn't even speak to his family?" Tess asked, still looking at Ernest.

"He has no family," Lily said quietly, then added so softly that Tess could barely hear her, "I don't think it's right to talk about him when he's right here, Tess."

"Oh yeah, you're right," Tess agreed, embarrassed. "So Annabelle and Lily are sort of like family to you, Dr. Finley?"

"Y-yes," Ernest answered without hesitation. He nodded at Tess, then dropped his head to study his hands. Lily and Tess stared at him, dumbfounded.

Tess looked past him and gasped. At the other end of the hallway two women were slapping each other. A nursing assistant was talking quietly to them, gently pulling the dominant woman away. Suddenly the dominant woman wheeled around and smacked the nursing assistant across the mouth just as the subordinate woman backed up and fell to the floor. She landed with her back against the wall and began to whimper. Tess sprang to her feet.

In the very moment she did this, her attention immediately shifted to Gloria Perez who sat less than ten feet away in her wheelchair pulling her shirt up over her head revealing breasts that sagged so low they rested on her waist. No one seemed to notice or care that Gloria sat topless while the nurse in the hallway examined the fallen subordinate woman. Tess shuddered almost audibly.

"Tess," Lily started, "Do you want to go?"

"What?" Tess tried to subdue the bewilderment in her voice. She sank into her chair, then turned to look at

Lily who still appeared totally unaffected by everything around her.

"Really. You should go," Lily said.

"I'm not supposed to be at this school. How will my mother find me?" a voice said behind her.

Surprised, Tess jerked around to see Doris hovering over her. Doris's head was tipped to one side, her expression a question mark.

"I'm sure your mother knows where you are," Tess told Doris, wondering if this was the right thing to say. Doris seemed unconvinced and glared at Tess, clicking her tongue.

"Tess, take my keys. Go home. Settle in. I'll call you in a while to come get me," Lily said, "Really. It's okay I just want to wheel Mother around the courtyard and spend a little time. I think she's enjoying having her dog here. Besides, I want to talk to Clancy. You know, the red-haired witch-nurse."

Tess suppressed the urge to snatch the car keys and bolt out the nearest exit. She glanced back at Doris who seemed to be waiting for an answer. Ernest was petting the dog while Annabelle chatted pointlessly. Gloria, still topless, had been wheeled away by Carlos, while the two slapping women in the hallway were beginning to square off again.

The red-haired witch-nurse was trying to change a bandage on the leg of a woman who was flailing her arms and kicking as she screeched broken curses. Someone had switched the radio on to a big band station, turning the volume up so loud that Tess could barely hear Lily giving her directions back to the house. Benny Goodman's band pounded through the dayroom. Residents began to wander aimlessly though the halls.

"Oh no. I'm fine, really," Tess shouted, then sighed, "Are you sure about this? Yeah, maybe I should go. If you're sure."

When she returned to the Storm's house, Tess plopped onto the sofa and inhaled deeply. She'd felt bad about leaving Lily behind, but she'd had enough. She was glad for the time to think. Lily needed help. For a moment, Tess considered calling Lily's ex-fiancé. The only reason they'd split up was because of Annabelle's persistent interference. Maybe he would want to know about Annabelle and how alone Lily was. Well, she wasn't all that alone. She had her friends, didn't she? Oddly though, most of Lily's best friends were in Minnesota. She had never let go of that. Her decision to hold on to the lake cottage had been unalterable. Selling her parent's Texas home had been automatic, almost a relief.

So, they would have to start the process of sorting through Stanley and Annabelle's belongings. An entire lifetime of possessions. As she thought of this, Tess remembered Lily telling her about the storage cartons in the attic. She specifically remembered the carton Annabelle had been looking through when she'd come across the old photo album. Was the album still there? Had Lily moved it? Or had Annabelle had a moment of clarity and hidden it?

There had always been something secretive about Annabelle. Tess's mother had told her that Annabelle was from a long line of straight-laced kooks one step away from the loony bin. Whatever her secrets were, maybe if Annabelle had revealed them before she'd succumbed to Alzheimer's, she perhaps could have let go of her stranglehold on Lily.

Tess climbed the stairs to the attic. She felt around for a light switch just as thin cord brushed the side of her head. She pulled on it and instantly the space around her was lit with a dim yellow light. The attic was filled with cardboard cartons labeled MISCELLANEOUS ITEMS just as Lily had described. She followed a narrow path to the far end. It was barely illuminated by the bare swinging bulb at the entrance. But there was no mistaking the carton Annabelle had opened. The contents were strewn into a swirl on the floor. Tess looked into the carton and saw Annabelle's photo album placed neatly on top of a pile of old curtains.

She looked through the photos slowly, marveling at this glimpse into Annabelle's past. All Tess had known of Annabelle's family was that they had lived at the uninhabited end of the lake where cattails invaded the shoreline. Tess's mother had told her that the Doyle's had no real friends and lived like hermits.

In school, Annabelle had been quiet, studious. She'd been considered brainy even. The other kids left her alone for the most part, calling her a bookworm. But then, in her last year of high school, she'd changed. There had been a new wildness about her that couldn't be explained. She was suddenly popular and overly social. Shortly after, she'd disappeared for a few years. The next time Tess's mother saw Annabelle, she was married to Stanley, a professor from the university. And there was Lily, their baby. They'd moved into the Doyle's lake cottage after Annabelle's parents had moved away and stayed until Lily was six.

Annabelle's past had only intrigued Tess because she had been so abusive to Lily. She hadn't been abusive in the traditional way with physical beatings, but psychologically and emotionally. But thankfully, Lily had her father. His great affection for her seemed to fill in the spaces left by Annabelle's defectiveness as a mother. Tess wondered if perhaps Annabelle had been jealous of this. But no, Annabelle was strong and decisive, secure in her marriage and in her ways. It had to be something else. Or maybe it was nothing. Maybe Annabelle truly was a straight-laced kook one step away from the loony bin.

Tess started to close the photo album when she was suddenly struck by a photo of Annabelle sitting on the hood of a car with two young men. She looked more closely, then sucked in a quick breath. One of them was Frank as a young man. Frank, the old guy from the hardware store back home. Frank, who showed up in the summer to work at the hardware store and spent all his evenings drinking and smoking at the local tavern. Frank, the ladies' man. Always on the make. A huge flirt. She'd started to notice him more after Lily had mentioned the photo album. Frank. Frankie. Of course. But what did it mean? Did it mean anything?

The cell phone in Tess's pocket rang, jolting her forward as though she'd been caught doing something wrong. She slammed the photo album shut and dropped it back into the carton as she snatched the phone from her pocket.

"Hello?"

"Hi Mom," Teddy sounded grim and too old for his years. "Everything okay down there in Texas? How's Lily? How's Annabelle?"

"We're okay, what's going on?" Tess wondered why her son would call so soon. She'd already let her husband know she'd arrived in Texas.

"Yeah, well, it's Dad. I'm not supposed to call you, but I am anyway. We had a big storm this morning and that giant cottonwood fell on the house right through the roof. Everyone's okay, but Dad hurt his back somehow. Maybe he thought he could move the tree off the house, I don't know. Now he's laid up and is going to move in with me here at the lake cabin and—" he stopped to take in a breath.

"Oh no," Tess groaned, "are you sure he's okay, Ted? I mean did he see the doctor yet?"

"Oh yeah, Will Larson took him over to Doc's office. Dad's fine," he went on, "Mom, can you come back? I mean—nothing against Dad or anything, but I'm trying to get ready for that big art show. I've got stuff everywhere. He's really in the way. And you know what a baby he is."

"Let me talk to him," Tess said.

"He's asleep. Doc gave him some pain pills. You want me to try to wake him?"

"No, no, forget it. Have him call me when he wakes up. I'll come back. You're going to have to put up with him for right now though, Teddy. Okay?" Tess said, her heart sinking. Lily had counted on her to help with getting Stanley and Annabelle's house ready to put on the market.

After they hung up, Tess reached for the photo album again. She held it to her chest without opening it, thinking about Frank and Annabelle, trying to make a connection. But she couldn't. They were two of the most dissimilar people she could imagine. She ran her hand through her mop of blond curls and shrugged as she dropped the photo album back into the carton on top of the curtains. But the album hit something hard under the curtains.

Reaching beneath the album, Tess tugged on the folded fabric. Slowly, she began to unfold layers of material to expose the object. When she got to the final layer, she lifted it out of the carton and let the curtain drop to the floor. She stopped cold.

It was the red box. Annabelle's red box. A small pine box painted red, but fading, the paint chipping away, locked with a small padlock. Tess stared at it, feeling as though she'd discovered the Holy Grail. She sank to the floor and placed the box in her lap.

Someone had painted it bright red a long time ago. It had been padlocked shut. Tess studied it. Just a faded red box. Big deal, she thought. But why was it locked? And why had Annabelle been so anxious to find it? To destroy its contents? Was that what she'd said? Tess had never paid much attention to Annabelle's whole quest to find the red box. It had seemed sort of ridiculous. Even fabricated. But now here it was. And what was she supposed to do? Bring it to Annabelle and tell her it had been found? Would Annabelle even remember now?

"Tess?" Lily's voice boomed up the stairs as the front door slammed, "Hey, where are you?"

Tess sat upright, her back straight against the carton, frantically trying to cover the red box with the curtain as she heard Lily bound up the stairs to the attic.

"Doris's son gave me a lift home. Tess?" Lily stopped short of her friend, trying to adjust her eyes to the dimness of the attic.

"Lily. I have it. I found it. I found the box."

"What box? What're you talking about?" Lily sat cross-legged on the floor next to Tess.

"Annabelle's red box. Remember?" Tess lifted the curtain from the box in her lap trying not to be too dramatic.

"'Whoa....look at that. So it does exist," Lily said as she leaned forward to look. "Did you open it?"

"Of course not! That would just be wrong," Tess said, "and I don't have the key anyway."

"Key?"

"It's padlocked shut."

"Of course."

"Lily, I know who that Frankie guy is now," Tess said suddenly.

"What Frankie guy?" Lily said.

"C'mon Lily, think back. The guy you told me about from your mom's photo album," Tess said.

"Oh yeah. That guy Annabelle was so weird to in the grocery store when we were in Minnesota," Lily said. "Who is he?"

"He's works at the hardware store in town every summer. His name is Frank," Tess said.

"Yeah—and?"

"And nothing. That's all. He's the same guy in these photos with your mom," Tess said, pointing to the carton behind her.

"So you don't really know anything about him," Lily said.

"I mean I know that he's the same guy in these pictures," Tess said in a defensive tone. "But no, I mean yeah, I don't know anything about him. Except that he's a drunk, I guess. He hangs out at the bar all summer. Picks up women. Probably in his fifties. Nice looking in a rough sort of way."

"So what do you think we should do?" Lily asked.

"About Frank?"

"No, no. About the red box. What should we do about the stupid red box?"

"Well, open it, of course, what else?" Tess said.

"Or should we take it to Annabelle?" Lily glanced at the box and shrugged.

"Lily, seriously, do you think Annabelle remembers it?" Tess asked, studying her friend's face.

"I'm going downstairs for a bottle of wine. We'll toast to the discovery of Annabelle's red box!" Lily said, suddenly festive. She sprang to her feet and sprinted down the attic stairway.

She returned in less than a minute with a bottle of red wine, two glasses and two pillows. They wasted no time in pouring the wine and clinking their glasses together in a toast to Annabelle and her secret red box. They drained their glasses and laughed as they settled onto the pillows.

"Where do you think she put the key?" Tess asked. She had finally moved the red box from her lap onto the floor between them. They watched it as though it would at any minute pull the curtain up around itself and slink away.

"Swallowed it. Annabelle probably swallowed the key a long, long time ago," Lily giggled as if this were hilarious. Her laughter faded when Tess didn't join her.

"Funny, Lily. Hey, do you remember how my mom taught us to drive that summer when we were twelve?" Tess said. "You plowed down the mailboxes and everything in your path, which turned out not to be the actual road."

"That was crazy," Lily said. "What made you think of that?" She poured more wine into their glasses.

"I don't know," Tess said, shrugging. "Something about that photograph of your mom sitting on the hood of the car with Frank and the other guy. They looked like just any other ordinary rebellious kids."

"Annabelle? Rebellious? Not likely. Good thing she never found out about your mom teaching us to drive," Lily let out a low whistle. "I mean, c'mon—I wrecked your mom's VW. I never could get that clutch thing right. She was so cool about it—your mom—really great. I'd always wanted her to be my mom instead of Annabelle, you know?"

"Did she ever hit you, Lily?" Tess asked.

"Your mother?" Lily said, shocked.

"No! No, silly. Are you drunk?" Tess said, now beginning to laugh, remembering how she and Lily could get drunk on the smallest amount of wine. "I mean your mom. I mean Annabelle. Did Annabelle ever hit you?"

"Sometimes. Usually she'd just slap me across the face when I least expected it," Lily said, gazing at the red box as if it were a sleeping Annabelle. She undid the band from her ponytail, letting her hair fall around her shoulders, brushing strands away from her face.

"I hate that. I hate that she did that to you," Tess said, folding her hands in her lap and staring at her laced fingertips. "Lily, I think Annabelle had problems. She never seemed all that happy to me."

"Really? But she and Dad were happy. They were inseparable. I figured I'd never find—well, you know—that kind of relationship—I mean, for myself," Lily said. Her words slowed between gulps of wine.

"But you and Kip—you guys were really compatible, Lily. You really should've set an immediate date after you got engaged. Why didn't you?" Tess said, tilting her head back to swallow wine straight from the bottle. She felt herself drift into Lily's past as though it were her own.

"We did. It's just that Annabelle kept coming up with reasons to change the date," Lily said. "I guess we should have eloped. I don't really blame him for walking away."

"Maybe you should call him. Or maybe I should. Do you want me to?" Tess said.

"No, he's married now or living with somebody or something, plays guitar in a band in his spare time, works as a master chef at some Austin restaurant." Lily closed her eyes and sucked in a slow stream of the musty attic air. "I've really no idea what he's doing. It's been three years. Anyway, you know me. Always ten steps behind what's really going on. I should've seen the end coming."

"So what do you think is in this box anyway?" Tess said, tapping the lid with the toe of her shoe.

"Nothing. Something. Who knows? I can't imagine that it could be anything so important," Lily yawned. "Annabelle said it was insurance papers."

"Boring. But what if it's a big wad of cash? What if it's a million dollars in gold?" Tess said, leaning forward to grab hold of the padlock.

"Please. Stanley and Annabelle Storm never had a big wad of cash stashed away." Lily rolled her eyes. "Now you're the one who's drunk."

Suddenly Tess stood up. She swayed slightly from the wine, grabbing hold of the carton. She peered inside, "The key is probably in here, Lily."

"Don't even bother looking," Lily rolled her eyes. "We can just pry the hinges off, can't we?"

"I don't know. With all that dried paint?" Tess examined the box, but her vision was swimming slightly. "Lily, I have to leave in the morning. I'm sorry. I hate this, but I have to get back to Minnesota. A tree fell on the house."

"Oh no! Was anyone hurt?" Lily said, sitting up straight.

"Sam's back is out. Who knows how he did that? But I told Teddy I'd be back," Tess said. "Will you be okay? I hate to abandon you. I can come back in a few weeks."

"No, no. You go. I'll be fine," Lily's voice was thin and uncertain. She dropped back into a comfortable slouch and stared at the floor.

"I'm so sorry, Lily. Maybe I should come back at the end of the week," Tess said.

"Wait a minute. Holy crap, Tess! It's not inside the carton," Lily said, suddenly alert. She shot forward on her hands and knees towards the base of the storage carton.

"What? What're you doing?" Tess said.

"Tess. It's the key. I remember now. Annabelle dropped it that day she was going through the photo album," Lily said as she slipped her hand under the carton and produced an old padlock key.

"Son of a—open it! See if the key works," Tess nearly shouted.

Lily slid the key easily into the lock and turned it, then stopped.

"What? What is it? Open it. Doesn't it open?" Tess said excitedly.

"I can't," Lily said, removing the key and closing her hand around it.

"What? It won't turn the lock?" Tess said suddenly exasperated, "Let me try it."

"No, Tess. Not you. Not me. I have to give it to Annabelle," Lily said grimly. Her expression became hard and distant.

"You cannot be serious. Annabelle won't remember—" Tess started, then stopped, realizing Lily was battling some internal conflict. She watched tears well up in her friend's eyes. She reached out to give Lily a hug, but missed. "You're crying? Why? What could possibly make you—?"

"I'm a tiny bit drunk. But even so, I know that I have to give Annabelle a chance. One last chance," Lily said. She slumped back onto her pillow, accidentally knocking the wine bottle over onto the floor.

The two of them watched as a puddle of red wine formed a tiny river that trickled towards the storage carton. They watched in silence as the carton soaked up the tiny spot of color. Lily began to laugh almost inaudibly. And then, as though watching an uproarious event unfold, her laughter turned boisterous. Tess stared at Lily, trying to grasp her friend's shifting emotions. Finally, she threw back her head and laughed, too, not caring why.

"The wind speaks
Through the quiet flutter
Of the poplar trees
Above abandoning
The slates of perfect illustration
While dusted clouds unleash
In graceful freedom and I
Exhale."
  —Diane Schonblom

CHAPTER 14

Lily

Ordinarily, a shift from blue and pink to tonal-colored flowers would have accompanied the passing of seasons at the Green Thumb Garden Shoppe, but this year, Lily had been slow to update the display of potted plants. It was nearly Thanksgiving, and there were still pink begonias on the tables mingling with the rust-colored chrysanthemum and pumpkin arrangements. It wasn't until a customer remarked about the clashing colors that Lily realized how dispassionate she had been about her store over the past months.

She hadn't even introduced a new line of ceramics created by a potter she knew from her poetry group. She'd stored everything in the back office during the summer and had simply forgotten it. Exquisitely crafted, colorfully glazed pots were covered in a thick layer of dust. Lily had to step over them nearly every time she entered the back office.

The assistant manager and store clerk were no help. They had tiptoed around Lily since the time Annabelle had slipped out of the shop into the street and become lost. Why had she hired such timid people? Lily wondered what kind of lives they must lead outside of work. But then, hadn't she hired them for their quiet, eclectic demeanors? They rode bicycles to work, sipped herb tea on their breaks and listened to flute music while they read beat poetry.

Lily sighed. A multitude of wind chimes hanging from the arbor above her head jingled and clanked in a kind of primitive melody. She closed her eyes and listened to the sound. All around her the pungent scent of freshly watered plants hung in the air. She dropped her head back into the antique rocker she had placed here for customers. It was a peaceful spot that overlooked rows and rows of native plants, grasses, flowers, a trickling pond and unusually sculpted birdbaths. She gazed through the arbor vines towards the evening sky, focusing her attention on a finch peeping through the door of one of the many birdhouses for sale.

The days were getting shorter and the store was beginning to dim with the approaching dusk. When the front door opened, Lily barely noticed. She didn't notice him until his dark shape loomed over her.

"We're closed!" Lily started, sitting upright, adjusting to the intrusion. She knew him. But out of context, and so abruptly, he seemed horribly sinister.

"I thought I might find you here. How are you, Lily?" he said.

"Kip?" Lily stood up, smoothing her hair into place. "What are you doing here?"

"What? Not even a hug?" Kip smiled, giving her a bear hug that knocked the breath out of her for a moment.

"Oh, now wait a minute—did Tess call you?" Lily reeled back on her heels, locking eyes with her ex-fiancé the way she'd done for so many years. He smelled like fresh soap and mint toothpaste. He had a beard, which was new. It made him look distinguished, like a scientist or a professor.

"And what if she did?" Kip said, "Would that be so bad? You should have told me, Lily. I mean, about Stanley. And, about Annabelle." He dragged a weather-beaten Adirondack chair across from the rocker and sat, pulling her along until she reluctantly sat beside him. The wind chimes jangled softly in a sudden breeze, tossing his mop of dark hair away from his face. His suit coat and khaki jeans made it seem as though he was dressed for a destination other than visiting her. He still looked youthful but wary with age. He had tiny lines at the corners of his eyes that had not been there the last time they'd seen each other.

"The beard is a good look for you, Kip," Lily said as she continued to study his face.

"You think?" Kip briefly stroked his chin, but then stopped abruptly and said, "Why didn't you tell me?"

"Why? What difference could it make, Kip? I'm taking care of her." Lily didn't trust her voice to sound capable. She looked down at her garden clogs, noticing dark water stains and greenhouse mud on the toes. Her faded blue jeans were ripped at the knees, her clean white shirt covered by a smudged Green Thumb Garden Shoppe apron. Her hair, which had been recently cut too short, was tied into a stunted ponytail. Her face was scrubbed clean of makeup. Self-conscious, she added, "You look great. Really great. How've you been?"

"Good. Been good," he said. Then as if reading her thoughts, "you, too. You look good, too. You've done a great job with the store." He looked around in the fading light as though it were the most interesting place in the world, his eyes finally settling on the row of birdhouses.

"So Tess told you that Annabelle has Alzheimer's disease, I guess." Lily switched on a lantern next to the bench. The light bathed them in sudden artificial tones. Hastily, she switched it off. "She's forgotten everything. Some stuff she remembers, I guess. She's different now. I don't know if it's the medicine they have her on or what. But she's sort of—I don't know—mellow, accepting. Even affectionate at times."

"Doesn't sound like your mom," Kip said as he reached across her and switched the lantern back on.

"For a while it was a living hell trying to keep up with her. She was obsessed with finding some red box and actually got hurt looking for it one time." Lily watched the tiny finch peek its head through the door of the birdhouse again. She felt fatigued and wasn't sure she wanted to talk about Annabelle anymore.

"So, did she find it?" Kip asked.

"Tess and I found it a long time after. It was padlocked shut." Lily remembered their discovery in the attic the month before. Remembered Tess's suggestion about calling Kip. Remembered she'd told Tess that it wasn't a good idea to call him. But seeing him now seemed natural and right as though little time had passed since they had split. It was just that she'd felt as though Annabelle's departure from reality needed to remain private.

"What was in it?" He seemed genuinely curious, which struck Lily as odd considering how utterly wretched Annabelle had always been to him. But then, perhaps since Annabelle had been rendered defenseless by her disease, he could look past all that and ask questions as though it really mattered to him.

"Don't know. I've never opened it." Lily closed her eyes and leaned her head into the back of her chair. "I gave it to Annabelle at the nursing home."

"So, was she glad to have it?"

"I put it in her drawer with the key one day," Lily said. "I thought if she sort of found it on her own that she would feel something like relief. I don't know. She's not really herself anymore. I don't know if she's found it or not."

"Seems like kind of a strange thing to do," he turned to look at her. He seemed to be scrutinizing her in the lantern light as though a rush of dark spirits from the past had suddenly surfaced.

"Not really. I think Annabelle should be able to discover it on her own." Lily felt suddenly defensive.

"Tess told me that Annabelle is really confused. She told me about her Alzheimer's friend. She calls him Stanley? The former doctor," he looked away as he said this, pity seeping into his voice.

"She's not that bad. She has good days and bad days, that's all." Lily pictured Tess when she'd visited Annabelle for the first time. Tess had been appalled. She'd wanted to get away immediately. "Besides, what does Tess know? She was only there the one time."

"You're still afraid of Annabelle, aren't you?" Kip's voice was low and careful.

"What? No! I'm not afraid of her." Lily stood up, suddenly angry. "Maybe when I was younger—I mean, yeah, Annabelle could be pretty menacing. I never knew what it was she wanted from me. I never knew why I wasn't ever good enough. Why I couldn't measure up to her. Why my choices were always wrong. Why she was so critical of my friends. Why she was convinced I was going to throw my life away. Why I would catch her looking at me sometimes as though I were about to step off the deep end into nothing and she—only she knew enough—or knew how—to stop me."

Lily realized her voice had escalated into a high pitched squeal. The more she spoke, the angrier and confused she became. She suddenly wanted Kip to leave. It irritated her that he continued to sit, staring straight ahead as though he might be able to solve the problem of Annabelle and Lily Storm in this one visit.

"Yeah, that was kinda it, wasn't it? Nothing was good enough in her eyes." He leveled his gaze at her.

"But it wasn't you, Lily. It wasn't me. It wasn't Tess. It was her. It was your mother. There was something she kept locked inside. Something that she's never told you. Something that made her want you to be someone you couldn't be."

"You hated her, I know." Lily sank into the antique rocking chair and covered her face in her hands, thinking of the time Annabelle had ruined their first dinner party at Kip's apartment. After devouring the delicious meal he had prepared, Annabelle openly mocked him for wanting to be a chef. Why would any man aspire to work in food service, she had said and laughed malevolently at him. He'd been crushed. His own mother had passed away when he was sixteen, and it had taken him a long time to find his way, only to be berated by his fiancé's mother at every turn.

"I did, actually. She was horrible," he admitted.

"I just keep thinking that there's going to be some way—some final way that Mother and I can forgive each other, you know?" Lily wasn't sure she even knew what she meant. "It's like I'm hanging on to this thread, waiting to exhale."

"That's completely nuts, Lily. Why would Annabelle need to forgive you?" he said.

"Because. Because, I turned on her, Kip. A long time ago, I told her that she was a disastrous mother, that I would never forgive her for her cruelty to me, that I would only ever love my dad. After I left home, I was cruel to her every chance I got. I said things. Did things," an unexpected sob escaped her throat. She shot forward out of her chair and moved several paces away when he reached for her. "No! No, you can't understand this. I ignored her birthdays, Mother's days. At Christmas I bought gifts only for Dad. I told her I hated her. Hated her. Didn't care if she lived or died. I didn't even go to the hospital when she had major heart surgery."

"She had it coming," he said, helplessly watching her as she paced.

"Oh god," she covered her face in her hands again, "maybe I am afraid of her. Do you think? Do you think I'm afraid of my mother? Even now?"

"I don't know what to say Lily," he stood slowly, his demeanor shifting. "I don't think I can help any more now than I did then. Maybe I should go."

Lily looked at him. Annabelle had hurt his feelings one too many times. She knew he didn't want to relive those shadowy memories. Suddenly Lily missed Kip. She missed how close they'd once been. But to reach for the closeness now would be like reaching across the night sky. It wasn't fair.

"So you're just going to take off. Just like that? Why did you come here, Kip?"

"I don't know. I thought things might be—I don't know—different now." He wouldn't look at her, "like maybe I could help this time."

"I have to do this myself. I have to be there for her now. There's no one else," Lily said, her voice turning cold, distant. "Mother and I have to forgive each other even though the reasons for things will never be clear."

"I hope you can do that," he said.

"Do you?" Lily answered icily, suddenly wanting her anger at Annabelle to settle on him like a residue of dust. Something touchable. Something she could see. Something she could trace the words *Lily was here* in or brush away if she wanted to.

"I'll call you sometime soon," he turned abruptly to leave. He walked into the dusk of evening without looking back, gently locking the shop door behind him.

"No you won't," Lily muttered as she slumped into the Adirondack chair where he'd been sitting and stared into space. She felt sullen, defeated. She wondered how it was possible that Annabelle could still impact their lives while locked in the confines of a deteriorating mind.

When Lily entered the Rainy Alzheimer's Center hours later, she was still thinking about the droop of Kip's shoulders, the collapse in his voice as he walked away. She knew there was no place for him in the panorama that had become her life now. He was too real.

Lily looked around the dayroom for her mother. Most of the residents were in bed except for the few who wandered aimlessly for hours after the sun set. She'd heard the staff call their renewed state of night confusion "sundowner's syndrome," and she'd imagined them as cowboys on horseback riding into town for an evening of drink and merriment at the local saloon. *The sun-downer's gang.* Ernest was usually one of them, but not Annabelle.

When Lily didn't see her mother with the sun-downer's group, she went to Annabelle's room. She had been considering opening the red box for Annabelle, or at least showing her that it was in her drawer. It surprised Lily to find her mother sitting up in bed talking to someone who sat in her wheelchair with her back to the door. Lily recognized the visitor immediately.

"Pearl! This is such a surprise," Lily said as she reached to grasp the cab driver's outstretched hands, "I never expected you to come by here. How nice."

"Please, girl. I come by here once or twice a week to visit with your mama and her doctor friend! We're all friends, ain't we?" Pearl winked at Annabelle, then beamed, looking from mother to daughter. She looked all dolled up as though she might have been dressed for church. "How're you, Miss Lily?"

"I'm okay, I guess. Hello Mother," Lily gave her mother a quick hug and began straightening her covers. "How nice that you have a visitor. Other than me, of course."

"Well, may the Lord bless you both. You been having a hard time with this?" Pearl's manner was as direct and straightforward as Lily had remembered.

Annabelle stared at the two of them without saying anything. Her eyes sparkled. She clasped her hands together like a child. She smiled a wide toothy grin that she would have considered unbecoming when her mind was still intact.

"No. Things are fine, you know. She's safe here. Comfortable, I think." Lily noticed Carlos walk by and waved at him, "Most of the staff is nice."

"Mmhumm, is that so?" Pearl narrowed her eyes and began rubbing her chin. "What I'm wonderin' is if you two have patched those differences of yours. You're not still mad at your mama, are you?"

"Mad? Oh no, no," Lily tried to laugh but couldn't, "She's different now. Sometimes she doesn't know me. Thinks I'm her sister, which is weird because she never had a sister. And then there's this," she said, opening the drawer to reveal the faded red box, "which is hers and was important to her at one time, but she's never opened it since I left it. At least I don't think she has."

"Probably she never opened the drawer, don't you think?" Pearl said.

Lily removed the box and placed it with the key on the bed next to Annabelle. Annabelle stared at it, her eyes widening. She looked like a child on Christmas morning with an unwrapped present. Lily couldn't be sure if her mother recognized it or not. She handed Annabelle the key.

"Is this mine?" Annabelle asked Pearl, running her hand along the top of the box.

"Well, I do guess so, sister lady," Pearl said.

"Do you want me to open it?" Lily offered, reaching for the key.

"No, no, no, you can't do it," Annabelle snapped, suddenly alert, wary, "It's mine."

"What's in it?" Pearl asked Lily.

"No idea. She'd been looking for it for months before she came here. One time she told me she needed to destroy its contents." Lily shrugged.

"Now here, sister lady. What if I open it?" Pearl suggested. Annabelle handed her the key without hesitation. Pearl glanced at Lily. She slipped the key into the padlock, unlocked it, then lifted the lid.

Annabelle reached both hands into the box and produced a photo, which she held at arm's length to examine. Lily could see it was a baby picture. After a moment, she realized it was of herself as an infant. It was a photo she'd never seen before.

"Big sister, baby Hazel," Annabelle said, still studying the photo.

"Looks like more photographs, some letters and some sorta book in there." Pearl peered into the open box and said in a low voice, "Looks as though your mama stored her earliest memories in this box."

Annabelle closed the lid and sighed. Still holding the baby photo in one hand, she placed her other hand firmly on the top of the box as though the memories needed to be contained. As though only one memory at a time could be examined.

"You're gonna need to go through all this with her," Pearl said, "You have to. You're gonna need to understand things about your mama. I just know it as sure as the sun comes up, that's all."

"I can't. It's her stuff," Lily said.

"Maybe. Maybe so. Don't matter," Pearl squared her jaw and took Lily by the shoulders, "I just know, you gotta do this. It's up to you. Somewhere, deep down, your mama wants you to know what's in here."

"Really? You think so?" Lily said, shocked. "How do you get that? I mean, she's always been so secretive. I just can't imagine that she would want me to—".

"Don't you ask me. Don't you even ask me how I know this," Pearl tipped her head, her expression becoming stern, unyielding, "Do you understand?"

Lily nodded. Pearl wasn't anyone important really. Just a cab driver that her mother had met at the height of her concealed confusion. But Lily had come to appreciate this woman for her strength and insight. It was as though she had some sixth sense about the things that only baffled Lily. And somehow, she had been right there each time Lily was stuck and floundering in a rut. She appeared long enough to give Lily a swift kick onto the right path, and then she was gone again.

"Okay. I'll do it," Lily said. She noticed Annabelle dozing off, the baby photo still in her hand. Lily lifted the box from the bed and cradled it in her arms. Annabelle continued sleeping, unaware. To Lily, her mother looked like a child, someone who needed protecting. Someone who had not been protected as a child.

It was late when Lily arrived home. Exhaustion overcame her as she stepped inside. Caesar greeted her at the door, yawning and thumping his tail against the door. She reached down to scratch his head, setting Annabelle's red box on the foyer bench. Tomorrow, she thought. Tomorrow Annabelle's memories can be set free.

*"Whipped sand and my footsteps
settle, I stand idle
in a melancholy trance. A loon
sounds out, small fish are dipping and I kneel
down, lay in the water, bare flesh
to earth, soul to God."*
— Diane Schonblom

CHAPTER 15

Lily

Lily opened the study window, letting the scent of dampened leaves drift into the room. She pulled her sweater closer to her, shivering at the slight chill of the November morning. The neighbor's cat was crossing the street with exaggerated stealth. She watched as the cat stopped at the curb to sniff a newly fallen leaf, then slip like a ghost into the gutter. There were no birds singing, no neighbor's dogs barking, no boisterous kids, no rushing cars in the street. It felt like a day of national mourning.

Lily dragged Stanley's oak swivel chair up to the desk and sat, resting her hands on the red box in front of her. So this was it, she thought. The sought-after red box. At one time, Annabelle had been obsessed with locating it, but as her mind faded so had her desire to find it. But then, maybe Pearl was right. Maybe Annabelle had wanted Lily to discover its contents. Maybe she had been trying to lead Lily to it all along. Still, it seemed so illogical. Why would Annabelle do that? And what could possibly be so important that she would remember it even as she succumbed to dementia?

Lily turned the key in the lock and lifted the lid to an array of old photos that were stacked on top of a bundle of letters bound together by a purple velveteen ribbon. Under the photos were a few clippings from newspaper articles. One of the articles had to do with an investigation about a man who had been found dead from what appeared to be an accidental fall from a balcony in Beau Lake. It was barely legible from being handled too much. Another article had to do with a young girl's drowning death. There were several clippings about World War II and a few others were book reviews.

She placed the photos and the newspaper clippings on the furthest corner of Stanley's desk, then glanced through the pile of letters. Most of them were written by Annabelle or Stanley with postmarks dating back more than thirty years. Lily stacked them on the desk next to the photos.

At the bottom of the box was a leather bound book filled with writing. The writing in the beginning of the book seemed juvenile. The lettering was chaotic with loops and swirls. Most of the early entries were a few sentences written by a child just learning to write.

The book was so threadbare that it fell open easily. Lily sucked in a deep breath. She felt as though she were intruding into the private space tucked deep within her mother's memory, a memory now ravaged by an incurable disease. She exhaled slowly, picked up the book and held it against her chest. Feeling suddenly burdened by the weight of its contents, she dropped it on the desk and stared at it. After a moment, she began to thumb through pages of childlike doodles comprised of abstract shapes and elementary school writing exercises until she came to the first of the longest entries. Annabelle had written in manic clustered spurts with gaps of time between entries.

"Okay Mother—what is so important—what is it you don't want me to know?" Lily whispered to the book in front of her.

Dear Diary,

It's May 29ᵗʰ today and I am now twelve years old. Mother told me that I am not to talk about it being my birthday though because it will make Father angry so I'm out here in the boathouse listening to the waves. Mother and Father never come to the boathouse. I believe they think it's haunted. Maybe because of all the loons. I heard a loon calling out in the reeds. It sounds lonely.

Yesterday, I heard Mother and Father arguing about my sister. They were talking about the day she drowned. Father kept saying that it was the only answer for such an evil child. Mother sounded as though she might have been crying but then Father yelled something at her and slammed his fist into the wall. It became so quiet after that I was afraid they might hear me outside their door so I had to sneak away.

My sister wasn't evil. I remember when she would tell me stories and sing songs to me until I'd fall asleep. She was very kind to me. I wish she was here. Maybe we would have a birthday celebration in the boathouse.

My face is swollen from where Father smacked me yesterday when I'd forgotten I'm not supposed to sing in the house. I was just humming a song we'd learned in school. I didn't even know Father could hear me. I thought I was being quiet. I'm not supposed to make any noise at all in the house when Father is home. I think my face might be bruised but Mother took all the mirrors away a long time ago, so I have to try and see myself in the water, if the waves will ever stop.
Annabelle Doyle

Dear Diary,

It's finally July. Summer is the best time to walk to the creek because it's so wild and overgrown. The trees are old and hang over the cattails in the water hiding the herons and ducks that live there. Some days there are deer drinking from the lake.

First thing I noticed today was a man fishing at the other end of the creek. I went over and talked to him for a bit and he showed me how to put bait on the fishing pole. He never caught a fish. Didn't seem to care. He talked to me about the Sioux Indians who once lived by the creek. He knows a lot about them and about all sorts of other history too, I think. I don't know how, but he already knew my name. He knew my mother and father. He gave me a book he had in his boat. He told me I could keep it. It's a book of poems called The Song of Hiawatha by Henry Wadsworth Longfellow. I hid it in the boathouse. When I went into the house, F shouted at me because I was supposed to be cooking supper but I guess I forgot because of the fisherman. After I made supper for Father (Mother had gone on to bed early, but then she got up and walked all over the house the way she does most nights), I was sent to my room with nothing to eat. I'm going to read the Hiawatha book in the boathouse tomorrow.   Annabelle D.

Dear Diary,

It's September and I'm back in school. It's Saturday today so I'm here at Cattails End trying to keep quiet in the house. Father had been drinking so much that when he lunged at me he fell flat on the floor. I only tried to tell him about the janitor job at school. It's not my fault he can't find steady work. Worst part is that I started to laugh at him there on the floor because I thought he looked stupid like that, so M made me stay in my room for a day and a half without food or water. I begged her not to but she wouldn't look at me or say anything. Her face was a blank mask. She just locked the door and went back downstairs like a ghost. I thought I'd heard her say she was sorry for me but she whispered the words so I don't know. I got so hungry by nightfall that I felt sick. Mostly I watched the waves splashing on the lake in the moonlight from my window.

The second day Mother made me recite the Ten Commandments to her through the door before she would unlock it. When she opened the door she peered around my room like she'd never seen it before. She asked me what I was doing locked in my room. She was angry at first. I didn't know what to say. Then she fell silent — completely silent. Her mask face reappeared. She came over and touched her hand to my forehead. She's never done that before. I thought she looked terribly pale, maybe sad, but she just turned away and was gone. *Annabelle Doyle*

Dear Diary,

The trees are all losing their fall leaves. It's fairly warm for an October day. I saw the fisherman again today at the creek. It has been a long time since the last time I saw him. I'd gone to wade in the creek to look for shells for my collection. The water was freezing. When I saw the fisherman I tried to hide the bruises on my arms from where Father had grabbed me but I couldn't hide the cut on my lip where Mother slapped me for something I can't remember. The fisherman didn't say a thing about it. It was like he didn't even see it. He asked me about the Longfellow book and I told him I had it well hidden and had read it quite a bit. He asked me questions about it the way school teachers do and I think I surprised him by answering everything correctly. I told him that I want to write important books when I grow up and he said he thought that would be splendid. He uses words like splendid and marvelous. He gave me another book. This one was about Sherlock Holmes, by Sir Arthur Conan Doyle.

The fisherman told me that his name is Dr. Dewey Storm but that I could just call him Dr. Dewey if I wanted. He told me that he had known my parents — mostly my father — for a long, long time and if I ever was in trouble with anything-anything at all, that I should contact him directly and he would see that I would get help. He said he was that kind of doctor. I don't know exactly what he was talking about. It seemed a strange thing to say but I agreed. He pointed to his house way far off *across the creek past the deer meadow by the tall pine trees. I'd never much noticed the house before. I wouldn't dare ask Mother and Father if they know him. They don't even know I go to the creek. Besides they've been working at the sugar beet factory most of the time now and don't pay much attention to what I'm doing. I'm thankful for that. AD*

Dear Diary,

It's March, still cold, not spring yet, but soon. Mother left suddenly yesterday with her sister from South Dakota. Sometimes Mother acts like she doesn't remember her own name. And her sister is as mean as a junkyard dog. Mother never said good-bye. They were just gone. I heard her sister say something about taking my mother to a Rapid City doctor which seemed to make Father furious. He started drinking early. He was supposed to be doing some odd jobs for Mr. Berg, but he probably thought it was too cold today to do anything except drink his whisky. I thought he might get angry at me for something and start hitting. When he shouts, he doesn't make a bit of sense. If I tell him I didn't do anything he just gets angrier. One time he made me stand in the snow with no coat for an hour. It was days before my bones felt warm again. Another time he made me eat a bowl of mustard. After the first three bites, I liked the taste of it but I acted like I didn't. Mostly he locks me in the little hall closet under the stairs for hours. I have to bend to fit in the space and I get tired after so long.

But today he never spoke to me even once. He just sat there, all blubbery and stupid. I tiptoed around him and he never even saw me. After I made his supper (which he scraped into the sink) and washed the dishes I went out to sleep the night in the boathouse under a hundred blankets and quilts. I was so cold, I shivered all night even though I'd lit a little fire in the wood stove. Father never saw the smoke. He never even knew I was gone from the house. I know that I could run away but where would I go?

Dottie Nelson from school told me I could come live with her one time back when we were eight, but she must have changed her mind because she doesn't talk to me too much anymore ever since Father got fired from her father's boat factory over in Beau Lake. A. Doyle.

Dear Diary,

It's April now. Not warm yet, but soon. I had a dream about my sister. She was running ahead of me, motioning for me to follow. I ran as fast as I could but as soon as I got close to her she disappeared into the water. I called for her but all I heard in reply were the waves slapping against the shore. And then M and F were suddenly in the water rowing a boat. I saw that Mother's hands were tied together with a rope. Father was rowing the boat so furiously that the water all around them formed huge whirlpools. He shouted my name, demanding that I step into the water and join them but I couldn't. I just couldn't. When I turned away, they were all of a sudden in front of me staring at me. When Father grabbed me by the hair and began to drag me to the water, I woke up. I woke up screaming in my bed but no one came. Mother and Father must have heard me, but no one came. And if they had, I might have screamed even more. Mother screams sometimes. Blood-curdling screams. I don't know why. Father locks her in the bedroom more than he used to. I hear her crying and walking in circles all day. She talks to herself but it doesn't make sense. It frightens me. AD

Dear Diary,

It's May 29th. My birthday. I'm 13 today. No one cares.

Dear Diary,

I am sitting at my window watching snow fall on the frozen lake. It's late November, the world is white and much too quiet except for the howling wind. Shouldn't a blizzard be even louder than a thunderstorm? It's so very, very cold. I'm wearing two sets of clothes. It's warm downstairs where M and F are. They have the wood stoves and plenty of wood. I know, since I'm the one who brought it in from the woodpile.

My teacher at school listens to me when I want to tell her just the simplest things but mother just wants me to leave her alone. She usually looks right through me as if I'm not even there. She tells me what to do and when to do it and screams if I don't do things fast enough. She misplaces things and then accuses me of stealing. I don't know what Mother cares about. She always looks either frightened or lost. When Father's anger is directed at me, Mother looks completely vacant. It's those times that I want to shake her — to make her see me. When she does see me, she doesn't seem to know me. She keeps repeating herself over and over until Father threatens her. This happens every day now. AD

Dear Diary,

Winter is over. Thankfully. The sun brings real warmth now. Happy 14th birthday to me. May 29th.

I went to the creek today. I saw that Dr. Dewey had another man with him. They didn't see me at first. I sat on the bank and watched the shapes of the clouds changing. Dr. Dewey and the other man weren't fishing anyway. They were just sitting in their boat talking. When Dr. Dewey turned and saw me, he waved at me to come over which I did. He introduced the other man as his son who is in college and had come home to visit. I think he said his name was Stanley. I couldn't think of anything to say because I felt like I had interrupted their conversation and the son just stared at me as though I'd dropped from the sky. Dr. Dewey asked me about how I'd been, how school was, did I need any more books to read. I told him everything was fine, that today was my fourteenth birthday. After I said that, he congratulated me. I didn't know what to say to that and by then I was staring back at his son because I'd noticed he had the same kind face as his father.

Dr. Dewey told me again to call on him if I ever needed anything.

I do.

I need to run away.

That's what I should have told him.

I need for someone to love me.
I wouldn't have ever said that.

                                        AD

Dear Diary,

I dread the coming of winter. It's only the beginning of October but still...

I woke up in the middle of the night because someone was standing over me. I barely took a breath because I was so frightened. I thought maybe I was dreaming but every time I shut my eyes tighter, the dream would not go away. I heard breathing and I recognized the smell of cherry-flavored candy. Then I knew it was Mother. I decided to pretend to be asleep. But then she touched my back and I jumped. I jumped so violently that I was suddenly standing beside the bed staring back at her. I was afraid to say a word or even breathe but I did my best to hide my fright because Mother is so unpredictable these days. All of a sudden, she turned and left the room without saying anything to me. When she had gone back downstairs, I closed my door and put a chair in front of it. I believe she was going to hurt me. I could see this in her eyes even though it was dark. AD

Dear Diary,

The winter has passed. It's April but it's still cold today like winter. And it's raining wet snow. It's been raining all day. When I went out to the wood shed to gather logs for the stove I nearly jumped out of my skin when an animal came from underneath the wood pile to sit beside my feet. It was a skinny little hound dog. Just skin and bones, poor thing. I sat down next to him and pulled my rain cloak over the both of us for a long time just petting him and talking. I can't imagine how he came to be out in the middle of nowhere down here by Cattails End. Maybe he'd come a long way. I had some bread from dinner in my coverall pocket (just in case M and F should lock me in my room for a long time with nothing to eat) and I fed it to him. He was so hungry. He followed me back to the house and I'm grateful no one saw him. I put him out in the boathouse for tonight. It's damp but better than being in the rain under the old wood pile. I'm going out there after M and F go to bed. They won't go to the boathouse so he can stay down there forever I expect. AD

Dear Diary,

I named the little dog Chance. I don't remember anybody ever being happy to see me the way he is. I brought him my food from dinner. He's quiet now.

Dear Diary,

It's been a month and Chance is healthier now. He's not skinny anymore. No one has discovered him yet. He never barks, never whimpers. I am able to sneak him out of the boathouse down to the creek without M and F knowing. He crosses his feet in front of him when he runs, like he doesn't know exactly what to do with all his happiness.

Dear Diary,

It's my fifteenth birthday but I wish I could die. I looked everywhere for Chance today. When I went out to the boat-house, it looked as though Chance had pushed the door open himself. There were scratch marks on the wood. I just know he was looking for me but M had sent me to town to the post office. I took the short cut so that I could get back quickly but a lot of the path was washed away from all the rains so I had to turn back. It took so long.

When I came back I saw that the boathouse door was wide open. I hid the mail I had with me in an old potato sack in the boathouse and went out to look for my dog. I was afraid to call for him because M and F would hear so I raced around all over until I finally found him under the wood pile. He'd been shot. I almost screamed out loud. I got down and put my arms around him and it was then that I knew he was alive. He was whimpering and really scared. I just know Father shot him. I just know it. I didn't know what to do so I stayed with him for a long time wiping the blood away from his neck. Then I remembered. Dr. Dewey told me I could call on him if I ever needed anything at all. So I picked up Chance and carried him across the creek, across the deer meadow, through the pine woods to Dr. Dewey's house. But I didn't get all the way there. Chance was so heavy for me. I finally stopped and put him on the ground. He could walk some, but I wouldn't let him. I sat there and cried harder than I ever have. Then I realized that someone was there. A shadow at first. After I shielded my eyes from the sun, I could see it was Dr. Dewey's son, Stanley. He sat down next to me on the ground and started to examine Chance kind of like a doctor would. Chance even wagged his tail a little.

Stanley asked me what happened and I told him I was sure my father shot him, that he was my secret dog. Stanley told me that the wound was superficial and that Chance would be okay after the wound was cleaned and he had a chance to rest up. He patted my arm and said it would be okay. But I said how could it ever be okay because next time my father might kill him. So he took Chance with him to help him get better. He told me I might come as often as I like to see my dog but he would be safer not going back with me to the boathouse. He said he would keep him for me for as long as I wanted, that Chance could sleep in their house by the fireplace fire. I hated to leave Chance like that. He whined when I walked away. I didn't know what else to do. I had to trust Stanley.

I saw Father's shotgun by the back door when I got back home. I'd had to stop to wash the blood off my hands in the creek. Father demanded to know where I'd been. I just told him that I'd had trouble getting home because the path had washed away from the rain. He stared at me as though he was waiting for me to say something about the dog. When I didn't say anything he lost interest in me.

I hope Chance will forgive me. As soon as I can get away with it, I'll go visit him at Dr. Dewey's house. AD

Dear Diary,

I promise I will not become like my parents. I want to be like Dr. Dewey. Educated and kind hearted. Father tells me that it's in my blood to be immoral and mentally ill. He says that someday I will have to keep my children boarded up in their rooms to keep them from fulfilling their destinies. Then he laughs. Mother starts laughing too. Except that Mother's laugh becomes shrill and she cannot stop until Father shakes her hard. Then she starts pounding on the table and crying. Nothing she says made sense. Her words don't come together right. I can still hear their laughter sometimes in my sleep. I wake up and want to scream. My parents aren't right. I know this now. AD

Dear Diary,

It's August now. School starts next month.

I went to Dr. Dewey's house today to see my dog but when I came to the edge of the deer meadow I stopped and sat on the cottonwood tree stump. From where I was I could see Dr. Dewey's son playing some kind of game with Chance. And they both seemed so happy. Stanley ran with Chance then tumbled to the ground. He was laughing and Chance's tail was wagging so hard it could have propelled him skyward. When Stanley tossed a stick straight up into the air, Chance bounced up like a pogo stick, trying to catch it in midair before it landed. The two of them rolled in the grass together, then sat side by side like best friends. Stanley seemed more like a young boy than a college man. I was a little embarrassed for him but then I think I felt jealous too. Chance was my dog. My best friend. I watched the two of them for so long that the light changed with the day's passing causing a glare and deep shadows, making it more difficult to see them. And then I thought maybe they might turn just so and be able to see me because the sun was shining on my side of the creek, so I turned and walked away. I just walked away. I don't know if I will go back again. I never had anything much to offer Chance. I'm afraid I don't have much to offer anybody. AD

Dear Diary,

I've not felt like writing for a long time.

Today, everyone is celebrating Christmas except for us.

I wonder where time goes when it flies away.

Maybe time is like the blue heron that rises up from the lake taking flight to a place of seclusion. Never to be seen again in the same way.

I'm sixteen now and I will be graduating early from high school next spring. I am first in my class. M and F don't know this because if I told them they'd just stare at me with their blank used-up faces. My teacher tells me that I have a promising future. She tells me that I can go to any college of my choice and that maybe I could become a teacher or even a professor, who knows? I did not tell her that I want to be a journalist. Maybe even a newspaper reporter. Or maybe a magazine editor. Or become a novelist. But of course, I cannot do these things. For one thing, poor girls don't usually have a chance of taking professions. How would I go to college? I have to care for M and F. Especially Mother, as she has become more and more remote. She is prone to fits of melancholy and rage and useless babbling. She doesn't know how to complete the simplest tasks. Sometimes she soils herself. Father is downright mean to her. And then she's mean to me. I cannot leave.

I have always believed my parents are somehow responsible for my sister Hazel's death. I wish Hazel could reach from heaven and tell me what happened to her in the end.

Tonight I believe I see her in the stars. AD

Dear Diary,

Spring is right around the corner and something fabulous happened today. An older boy, really handsome, followed me out of the grocery in town. At first I didn't pay much attention to him except that I knew he wasn't from our town. He looked like some Hollywood star. Like the type of boy M would make me cross the street to avoid. I stepped aside so that he could pass but he stopped beside me. He slouched up against the storefront and lit a cigarette. He asked me my name and some

*other questions. Every time I answered him, he'd look away
as though he didn't really care what my answer was going
to be. But if I tried to leave, he'd turn and stare at me with
the most piercing brown eyes I've ever seen. It made me feel
almost grown up. Which I am. I am grown up now. He said
his name was Joey. He only smiled once when I said something
that didn't come out right. But that one smile was enough for
me. I just wanted to know where he came from and when he
would be coming back. But he got into a convertible car with
another boy and sped away without saying good-bye. He's
nothing like the boys at school. He saw me differently. He
doesn't even know my family either. Maybe I'll see him again
someday.   A. Doyle*

Dear Diary,

*I overheard some of the girls at school talking about
Joey. They were acting ridiculous, batting their eyes and
giggling. They were saying that he'd only just moved here
from out of state. That he's a rich, fast boy who is gorgeous
enough to be a Hollywood star like James Dean. When I spoke
to Dottie Nelson about him later I told her that he had talked
to me at the grocery store in town before. At first she didn't
believe me. But then she told me I ought to stay away from
him. She told me that he is very bad. Dangerous even. When
she said the word dangerous she smiled. I cannot imagine
what she meant. AD*

Dear Diary,

*When I left school today, Joey was standing across the
street waiting for me. Me. I couldn't believe it. Dottie Nelson
whistled under her breath when she saw him and then almost
fainted dead away when she saw me go over to talk to him. I
almost didn't. But he was watching me. Watching me walk
out of the building. And he smiled a little. So I asked him
what he was doing there. He just shrugged and asked me if I
wanted to go for a ride in his convertible. Would I? Was he
kidding? I jumped in and rested my head on the back of the*

seat, feeling completely free from all the things that hold me down. He just laughed at me. Actually threw his head back and laughed. He drove me all the way to Beau Lake. I never cared that M and F might see that I wasn't home after school. Besides Father works late at the factory every day while Mother is locked in the downstairs bedroom. They never know if I'm upstairs. Half the time I'm in the boathouse anyway.

Joey told me things. He told me that his parents are wealthy Sicilians from Chicago who are always traveling so he and his older brother Frankie stay alone most of the time. He told me he dropped out of school to become an actor. He said he likes to live on the edge of the world, that nothing scares him. He said that he won't let anything ever take away his freedom. Nothing will ever tie him down. Never, he said, not ever. I know he meant it like it was the most important thing in the world to him. I just don't know what he means exactly.

I barely listened to his words anyway. Mostly I watched him say them. AD

Dear Diary,

Joey has come by every day for weeks now after school to whisk me away in his car. He drives me to his parent's home in Beau Lake. His parents are never there. It's almost as though they don't exist.

I believe I've fallen for him. But Dottie is right. He is fast. Too fast — he doesn't take no for an answer. But maybe if I can make him fall for me too he'll take me away from Cattails End for good someday. Some place where Mother and Father can never find me.

Once in the middle of the night Joey came to the boathouse, knowing he'd find me there. I told him to go because if Father found out that we were together, he'd likely shoot him on the spot, but Joey just shrugged and told me he could take on my drunken Father any old day. Nothing scares Joey. Nothing.

My grades are beginning to drop. I'm failing some courses. I won't graduate this year if I don't bring my grades up. My teacher tried to keep me after class to discuss it but I told some lie and left before she figured it out. I don't care about my grades anymore. What good is school going to do me anyway? The only way out is through Joey. AD

Dear Diary,

It's my seventeenth birthday. It should have been a good day but it was horrible.

After school, Joey's brother Frankie met me. I said, where's Joey? He said that Joey wasn't with him. He said he wanted to talk to me about something so I went with him. I couldn't imagine what he'd want me to know. Frankie's a nice boy. Good looking but nothing like Joey. We drove for a long time before Frankie spoke. Finally he told me. Joey is gone. Frankie told me that Joey took off on his motorcycle to another town where he has another girlfriend. He told me Joey has still other girlfriends too. I told Frankie I didn't believe him and why was he telling me all this? He said that he thinks I'm a good kid, but young, way too young to get mixed up with his brother.

I noticed he was chain smoking Lucky Strikes so I took one from the pack and lit it. I nearly threw up from the sensation of it but I wanted him to see that I can be just as wild as Joey. When I told him that Joey loves me, he started to laugh but then he looked over at me and quit. He stopped the car, got out and I followed him down the road. He shouted that I should stay away from Joey that he's wanted by the law in some town outside of Chicago for something violent, that he beat up a prostitute pretty bad. A prostitute? He told me Joey has a mean streak, meaner than my father's. And that when he's drinking, he loses all control. He said that he might hurt me someday too.

I was mad. Mad at Frankie. I smacked him across the face for all his lies but he just stood there. He kept on saying that I was too pretty, too smart, and too young. It didn't make any sense. Why would he lie like that? I cried in the car all the way back. Thankfully Frankie kept his mouth shut. He drove me back to Cattails End but not so close that Mother and Father would see us. I walked the rest of the way. I felt sick. I threw *up on the path several times. I feel horribly betrayed. I don't know if I feel betrayed by Frankie or by Joey. I don't know. I just do not know. AD*

Dear Diary,
It's been eighteen days and I still have not seen Joey. I daydream in class but after class I seem to be the center of attention. I get invited to parties and boys ask me out. This has never happened to me before.

I don't care. It doesn't matter. I feel sick every morning when I wake up and think of Joey gone. Gone off with some other girl. I saw Frankie in town one day but as soon as he saw me he started walking the other way. He can't face me. I can't face him.   A. Doyle

June 1st
At home, I had to clean. Mother gave me a brush a little larger than a toothbrush and told me to scrub the floors. At least I think that's what she said. A lot of her words are intense gibberish. Halfway through she stopped me and handed me a handful of bread dough. Just when I figured out that she wanted me to bake it she demanded I clean every window in the house. She couldn't remember the word for windows, kept using some other made-up word. So I started washing windows. Upstairs and down. While I did this, she paced and mumbled to herself. I tried to listen to what she was saying but it was just random words. After I finished the windows, I saw that she was lugging furniture around and when I stopped her she clearly told me that she wanted me to move the bedroom furniture into the living room and the dining room furniture into the spare bedroom. I didn't dare question her — she seemed possessed by demons. And lately she can become violent with no warning. She's strong. Insanely strong. I don't know which was more exhausting. Trying to follow her instructions and stay clear of her wrath or the physical labor of doing point-less work. I'm not sure at what point I passed out but when I woke up I was sprawled out on the living room floor — mother

was nowhere to be seen and Father was standing over me
telling me to get up. When I wouldn't, he kicked me with
his boot and told me to move all the furniture back where it
belonged. So I did it. Mother was sound asleep on her bed. I
felt weak and dizzy.

When I went up to my room later, it dawned on me. I'm
pregnant. Pregnant. God help me. I have to find Joey. No
matter where he is, I will find him.   A. Doyle

Lily closed Annabelle's journal. She reached for
the stack of letters, but stopped. It was too much. Too
much to absorb. Sadness began to well up inside her
like nausea. She covered her mouth with her hands. Her
eyes watered without the emotion of crying. Annabelle
pregnant at seventeen? Was Joey her father? Did Stanley
know this?

She'd never met Annabelle's parents. Annabelle had
never mentioned them. It was as though they had never
existed. Lily wanted to despise them, but she only felt
cold shock. Her grandfather had been a mean bastard
but her grandmother—her grandmother had been
what? Crazy? Or, Lily dreaded to think, did her grandmother have undiagnosed early onset Alzheimer's? It
was something no one knew much about in those days.
It made sense. It was the genetic type. Of course.

Lily turned to study her own pale reflection in the
window and shuddered. Her image in the glass dissipated as she focused her eyes on the neighbor's cat who
was now sitting complacently on the sidewalk gazing
back at her.

"Hope is the thing with feathers
That perches in the soul
And sings the tune without the words
And never stops at all"
— Emily Dickinson

Chapter 16

Annabelle

Nearly twenty years had passed since the day Annabelle moved away from her parent's home on Cattails End to live her life with Stanley, and yet the memory of that time never left her. It was like a hard knot balled up in the pit of her stomach that made her want to plunge into freezing water and swim against the current until her breath rushed out in icy gasps. Even as she imagined doing this, the feeling would burrow into the tiny fissures and cracks of her mind, slowly seeping into every surrounding cell until she had to give in, let go and brace herself for the next wave.

Other memories faded. Like summer at the lake. They came, they went, in and out, swept away by the breeze of a new season. But not this. Annabelle had forgotten a lot over that time, but not this. Never this.

The terrace where she sat had darkened with the vanishing of daylight. Stanley would be home soon from the British Literature class he taught on Tuesday evenings. Annabelle glanced down at the letters in her lap. She would need to put them away. Why had she read through them again? It wasn't as though she could change anything that had happened. Stanley would tell her to burn them. Burn everything, burn it all, he'd say. She'd replayed this over and over in her mind. Why couldn't she do it? It sounded so utterly simple when he said it.

Or was it because of Lily? Annabelle always thought that if she could just find some one flaw in the mechanism of her memory, some one thing that would show her that it had not happened exactly the way she remembered it, that she could face her daughter. She could rise out of the icy current and clutch Lily to her like a new beginning. They could begin again and this time Annabelle would welcome the tiny infant who screamed, red faced and hungry to be held.

But it wasn't to be. Reading the letters only caused her to feel even more detached. Stanley understood this about Annabelle. He alone had always been there for her. He had kept her injured dog when she was fifteen. He had kept her safe from her father when she was seventeen. He had kept her secrets about her mother. He had respected her pain. He'd never told anyone about her past. Not even Lily. Not even when he believed it might end the war that raged between mother and daughter.

Annabelle buried her face in her hands, rubbing her eyelids with her fingertips. She felt soothed by the damp hot air of early summer on her skin and the chorus of cicadas surrounding her. It was nearly dusk, but she could still make out the words on the pages of the letters. She smiled at this, thinking maybe it was just that she'd read them so many times she'd memorized them. She smoothed the paper with both hands and sighed heavily. She gazed up at the lavender sky of early nightfall.

A police siren wailed in the far distance. Annabelle listened to the sound until it vanished into the atmosphere. Should she have called the police that night? How would her life have been different if she had? She'd only run because she was scared, but what if she'd called the police to report—to report what? That she'd had a violent argument with her boyfriend who was so unspeakably drunk and so precariously close to the edge of the balcony that shoving him off had been as easy as dropping a rag doll to the concrete? That he had turned away just enough that he hadn't see her lunge at him? That the top rung of the balcony gave way against the sudden crash of his weight?

It was true his vision was so blurred that his reactions had become seriously impaired. And that was just it. He had been so drunk that in Annabelle's fury, she'd confused him with her father for a split second. It was in that split second that she saw only the color red. She saw red when she shoved him with every bit of force she could muster. She saw red when she heard the balcony rung give way, red when she heard the awful sound of his skull smashing against pavement. Red, as she bolted down the flights of stairs to the street. Red, as she raced to the highway. Red, as she hitched a ride home from Beau Lake with vacationers who were passing through. And red, as she sank to the floor of the boathouse and curled into a fetal position.

She'd had to find Joey to tell him she was pregnant. And to tell him that he absolutely must marry her. He'd swaggered toward her and locked his hands around her neck, his handsome face contorted with anger and all he said was, *never*. Floodgates opened and he shouted that she was nothing but a tramp, that he was not the father and that he would kill her like an insect before the bastard child was even born. When she'd started to sob, he laughed as loud and as maliciously as her father had the time he'd told her that her children would inherit her family's mental illness.

And for the tiniest moment, she saw her teacher's face, full of concern and disappointment, asking *why*

*have you thrown it all away? What have you done Annabelle?
How could you have been so stupid? Joey doesn't love you just
because you love him. Your parents don't love you just because
you are their daughter. Your mother doesn't care about you
just because you want her to.*

They were all monsters. They'd ruined her and they
didn't care. Now she would never amount to anything.
And her baby? The poor thing would never be right in
the world coming from such ignorance and violence
and to a mother who had absolutely no desire to raise
a child.

Annabelle had murdered Joey. It was murder. Or
maybe it was manslaughter. What was the difference? It
was the kind of act that was full of rage laced with insanity. Would she have gone to prison for life? How many
times over the years had she considered turning herself
in? How many times had Stanley stopped her, telling
her that she had been a tragic product of an abusive
home? Telling her that the real Annabelle was still in
there, waiting to surface, waiting to blossom.

And so, it had been concluded by the authorities that
Joey's death was an accident. He was an unruly boy out
of control, drinking heavily, too close to the edge of the
balcony of his parent's home, which evidently had a flaw
in its design. No one who knew him even questioned
it. Not his parents who had been abroad on vacation at
the time, not even his brother Frankie.

Annabelle lurched forward at the sound of footsteps
behind her.

"Didn't mean to startle you, sweetheart." Stanley sat
on the porch swing next to her.

In the dimness of evening, she couldn't make out
his face. It made her uneasy as though she was peering
into the past, or into the future when she and Stanley
might sit here as a docile elderly couple content just to
admire the flowers in the garden or the clouds in the sky.

Relieved that the years had passed so uneventfully. Relieved that their only regret was the flawed relationship between Annabelle and Lily. The important thing was that they'd kept Lily on track. She was in college now, majoring in journalism, following the dream Annabelle had to abandon. Lily was strong and bright and could handle her life without becoming dependent on anyone who might mistreat her. And wasn't that all that Annabelle had hoped for? She had been unable to love Lily from the moment her daughter was born. She believed in her heart that her daughter was defective because of her genes. Lily had the same willful, the same whimsical temperament as Annabelle.

"No, you didn't startle me," Annabelle said as she tucked the letters under the swing's cushion so he wouldn't see them. "How was your class?"

A strong breeze stirred the garden flowers, lifting the wind chimes Lily had given them into a tinkling melody. The smell of fresh cut grass filled the air around them.

"Good. It was good." If Stanley noticed the letters, he gave no indication. He seemed absorbed with thoughts of the day, of teaching his students at the university.

They listened together as the neighbor's dog began to bark in rapid succession at some unseen thing. A disembodied voice called to the dog and the barking quickly stopped. Stanley put his arm around Annabelle despite the heat of the evening. He smelled like a mixture of sea salt, old textbooks and fading cologne. Annabelle rested her head against his shoulder.

She hadn't loved Stanley when they'd first married so many years ago. When her father gave his permission for her to marry Stanley, he didn't know Annabelle was pregnant with Joey's baby. Her father hadn't cared. He had only imagined that somehow there would be money in it for him if his daughter married into the Storm family of doctors and professors. Annabelle's feelings for Stanley had grown gradually. Now she could not imagine her life without him.

She couldn't imagine what her life may have become if she hadn't run to Dr. Dewey Storm that awful night after she'd shoved Joey to his death. He hadn't even believed her at first. She was a petite girl, Joey was a well-built boy. How was that even possible? But Dr. Dewey promised to help her. She'd told him about the pregnancy, how she wanted nothing more than to end it, to make it stop. How she only wanted to return to school and make something of herself. Dr. Dewey told her he would find a way. But when Stanley returned from college a few days later, everything changed. Stanley wanted to protect her, *till death us do part*. He was determined. Somehow, he already loved Annabelle. Maybe he had always loved her. Maybe it would be enough. Maybe Stanley in his infinite patience could raise the child while she watched.

"Sometimes, I wonder…" Annabelle whispered, her voice trailing off. She noticed that the moon had begun to climb into the darkened sky spilling white light in its path, enough that she could see her husband's features more clearly.

"Wonder what?" Stanley stretched his legs in front of him, tipping the swing forward slightly.

"Oh well, I just wonder why the moonlight makes everything look as though it's washed in blue," she said, changing the subject in her own mind.

"You seem sad," he said.

"I am, a little."

"What is it?" The concern in his voice was immediate as though he expected any day for her to tell him that she regretted marrying him after all.

"I don't know. I was just thinking about my mother." Annabelle gazed up at a small cloud dancing across the full moon. "It was sixteen years ago today that she killed herself. Do you suppose if I'd been there for her, that she might—"

"No," Stanley said simply. He hated talking about the past. He'd always told her to think of the past as the rearview mirror of a car barreling forward in time. After a while, there is nothing left to see in the refection. "Your mother was an extremely troubled woman, Annabelle. She was—she was demented. Had been for a long time."

"You're right, I know." She felt a tiny well of desperation stir inside her, "you're always right. You can't ever leave me, do you understand?"

"More likely you'd leave me," he said. She could tell he was smiling without even looking in his direction.

"No, really. Promise."

"Promise," he laughed lightly, not realizing she was asking him to promise not to die first and leave her behind.

"I who had been afraid of the dark at night
as a child here in this room,
even when I lay safe by my mother's bed
now without fright watched here alone
until the break of day
my mother lying in the last sleep of all."
— Sister Maris Stella

CHAPTER 17

Clancy

"Are you as mixed up as we are?" the tiny white-haired woman asked, tapping lightly on Doris's shoulder. Doris was clinging to the nurse's station as though it were the railing of a turbulent ship. The small woman who peered into Doris's face was part of a chain of elderly women holding hands as they strolled through the Rainy Alzheimer's Unit.

"Oh no—I am not mixed up," Doris answered indignantly. "I am trying to get the keys to my car so I can get home." She eyed the small woman suspiciously, then dismissed her with an exaggerated jerk of her shoulder. She turned back to the desk where Clancy sat buried in charts.

Clancy glanced up at the women surrounding the nurse's station. None of them were aware that it was 6:15 in the morning or that it was Thanksgiving Day. They were still shuffling around in their pajamas except for the already-dressed Doris who now glared at Clancy without blinking. Apparently she was convinced she could bend Clancy to her will. Clancy smiled, thinking how Doris's state of dementia had barely changed since the day she had been admitted four years before. Doris was still looking for her car keys or the bus or her way home or her mother. She was still mixed-up.

"*Bueños Dias,* Happy Thanksgiving!" Carlos' voice boomed from the doorway. Just as he entered the secured unit, Ernest Finley darted out the open door, but was caught mid-motion by Carlos' strong grip. "Oh no you don't. Too early for all that. Let's not have that today. Okay, Ernest? *Por favor?*"

Clancy watched as Ernest turned and walked away. It amazed her that he still believed there was somewhere else he had to be.

"You're late, Carlos," Clancy shook her head. "And— please call him *Doctor* Finley. Why can't I get anybody to do that? I mean, how hard is that?"

"I thought you were spending Thanksgiving with your cousins in Dallas." Carlos ignored her irritability as he slouched against the nurses' station. He locked arms with Doris who gaped at him with wide-eyed curiosity. It was as though she was seeing him for the first time despite the fact that she saw him every day. She tilted her head back to flutter her eyelashes at him.

"Changed my mind. My cousin's house is too crowded with people dying to pass judgment on me. My persona would be totally blotted out. Besides, Mariama called in sick, so—"

"Really? She never calls in. What's with her?" Not waiting for an answer, Carlos glanced down the hallway in the direction of Annabelle Storm's room. "Hey, how's Annabelle doing?"

"Not well," Clancy's face clouded with concern. "I feel sorry for her daughter."

"So Annabelle's back from the hospital? Was it her heart condition?" Carlos still looked in the direction of Annabelle's room. Suddenly raising his eyebrows, he turned back to face Clancy, "Hey, wait a minute—you feel sorry for her daughter? I thought you hated the daughter."

"I did. I do. Or, I don't know exactly. I just don't get her," Clancy said.

"What's to get? Why do you have to analyze these family members anyway?" Carlos asked.

"I don't analyze family members," Clancy snapped.

"Always. You always do this." Carlos ducked as though her sharpened words might make physical contact with him.

"Not everybody. Annabelle's daughter has just always irritated me. I can't pinpoint what it is," Clancy began to twirl the ends of her hair. She stood up from the desk and looked past Carlos down the hallway. "It's just that she's so detached. She seems, I don't know, overly critical or something."

"So you don't like her because she reminds you of yourself," Carlos rolled his eyes. "Please. That's all it is."

"That's not true. Where do you get that?" Clancy glared at him even as she considered his words. "It's like I want to ask her why she even comes here. I've never seen her hug her mother. When she leaves, she barely says good-bye. She just seems like some sort of wooden puppet devoid of emotion. Annabelle gets more warmth from that other woman who comes to see her."

"What other woman?" Carlos folded his arms across his chest and began watching the other residents wander aimlessly around the dayroom. Clancy noticed that his hair was still wet from showering and that his aftershave smelled like insecticide. The blue scrubs he wore looked as though they had been professionally ironed.

"Oh, you know—she drives a cab. What's her name? Pearl? It's like she absolutely adores Annabelle."

Clancy thought of how Annabelle's face would light up when Pearl came to visit.

"Oh yeah, I know her," Carlos said, "the black woman with all the bracelets and rings. She's here every week. Did you know she always visits Ernest, too?"

Before Clancy had a chance to answer, one of the other nursing assistants yelled for Carlos from a room at the end of the hallway.

"Carlos! We need your muscles down here to help lift Claude!" The assistant popped her head out the door and added, "You just gonna stand around and gab all morning? What ya think? It's some sort of holiday?

"And a happy Thanksgiving to us all," Carlos snorted under his breath to Clancy, then started towards Claude's room.

Clancy watched him walk away, wondering why she didn't find his argumentative jabs at her more offensive. She noticed that he stopped beside Annabelle's room to wave solemnly at someone. He spoke a few words into the room, then continued to the end of the hall where the nursing assistant was now standing outside the room, her hands on her hips, tapping her foot.

It would still be dark for another hour. As far as Clancy could tell, no light was coming from Annabelle Storm's room. She couldn't imagine who Carlos saw from the hallway unless it was a coworker. She closed the chart she was working on and began walking in the direction of her patients' rooms.

Clancy moved soundlessly in and out of rooms, making short assessments of each resident still in bed. Gloria Perez awoke with a start and began cursing in Spanish. She made a fist at Clancy, and then closed her eyes, her head sinking deeply into the oversized pillow. She was instantly asleep, her hand still balled into a fist.

Annabelle's room was dark except for a dim lamp on the bedside table. Clancy squinted against the blinding hall light. She saw that Ernest was sitting quietly in the shadows on the bed opposite Annabelle's. The divider curtain partially hid someone who was talking in a low voice. It was Annabelle's daughter.

Lily was sitting on the chair next to Annabelle's bed with her back to the door. Her head was bowed slightly. There were wadded tissues at Lily's feet and on the bed. She held Annabelle's hands in hers while balancing a small open box of some sort in her lap. Annabelle was watching her daughter attentively. Lily's words came out in choked sobs.

Clancy instinctively began to back away. Something was wrong. Some terrible private matter between Annabelle and her daughter. Something awful, but something important. Something that was absolutely none of Clancy's business.

"Why, Mother? Why couldn't you have let Dad tell me? I needed to know," Lily sobbed.

Clancy froze in her steps. Instead of turning, closing the door and tiptoeing away, she held her breath and stepped softly into the room. Ernest turned to look at her. She inwardly panicked, hoping he would not give her presence away. But he said nothing. She exhaled slowly.

"It's not fair. I'm so, so sorry. Can you understand at all?" Lily pleaded. Her sobbing was accompanied by tiny hiccups. "I would have been okay knowing. At least I would have understood everything better if I'd known how cruel your parents were to you."

"And about your mother?" she continued, "She must have had this same illness. And what will happen to me? And what if I have kids? There's a genetic risk, Mother. Dr. Mason told me about early onset—"

Annabelle reached out her hand and touched her daughter's hair. Her eyes glistened. It was hard for

Clancy to tell what emotion she saw on Annabelle's face.

"Hazel?" Annabelle said clearly. She smiled and put her hand under Lily's chin.

"No Mother. Not Hazel. Not your sister. It's me, Lily. Your daughter." Lily patted her mother's hand, waiting for some spark of recognition in her eyes.

"Lily." Annabelle repeated. She turned to look at Ernest then turned her eyes back to Lily, "sister."

"Daughter," Lily corrected.

"Daughter," Annabelle said finally. She closed her eyes and sighed.

"I was horrible to you. Mean and cold and unbending. I was hostile. I didn't understand anything, Mother." Lily had stopped sobbing. Her voice was stronger, more determined, "I had no idea you had been through so much heartache and trouble. I had no idea how hard you tried to be mentally normal. I just thought you hated me. I didn't know about any of it. I would have been a better daughter. I would have been more supportive. Especially over the last several years."

"Well, now, now—now. Everything's—fine." Annabelle seemed perplexed but receptive, curious.

Clancy's eyes had begun to adjust to the darkened room. She saw that Lily had spread old photographs across Annabelle's bed. The box that sat in Lily's lap held an opened book and letters. It seemed odd that Lily had done this since Annabelle took no interest in any of it.

"Dad was good to me. He will always be my dad, you know," Lily began again to quietly sob. "What happened to my real father was an accident. You couldn't have known what you were doing. You'd been through too much. It wasn't your fault. You managed to keep it together all these years. How could you not look at me and see all the terrible things that happened to you? You had no idea how to raise a child. And I never made it easy. I understand all that, Mother. I know Dad and Grandpa Dewey helped you manage over the years. It's not a matter of me forgiving you. You did as well as you could. It's me who should ask for forgiveness."

It was too many words. Annabelle shuddered slightly. She took Lily's hand and held it to her face. Silence fell on the room like a veil. Even Ernest made no sound. Clancy willed herself to stop breathing long enough for the moment to pass.

"I love you, Momma," Annabelle finally whispered, her eyes still closed. A single tear rolled down her cheek.

"It's Lily," her daughter corrected, then added, "I love you, too."

"Lily," Annabelle repeated. Suddenly she reached forward and embraced Lily.

"Can you forgive me?" Lily pleaded, "Can you ever forgive me?"

"Yes," Annabelle whispered. "I love you, Momma."

Lily dropped her head onto the bed. Her sobbing became uncontrollable. Tiny tremors shook her shoulders. She seemed frail suddenly, almost childlike. Ernest got up from his place on the other bed and stood behind her not knowing what to do. He reached out to touch Lily's head but left his hand suspended in air until it drifted back to his side. Annabelle's eyes were closed, her breathing became more ragged. Clancy heard footsteps in the hallway behind her.

"Clancy—" Carlos started, "Where are you?" His voice boomed across the corridor. Lily jerked her head up and turned just as Clancy slipped out of the room.

"Shhhh, what do you want?" Clancy hissed.

"What're you doing anyway?" Carlos asked without lowering his voice. He looked from Clancy to Annabelle's room, then back to Clancy.

"Nothing! What do you want, Carlos?" It was at that moment Clancy realized she'd been crying. She began furiously wiping at the tears on her face.

"What is it? Is she dead?" Carlos whispered, suddenly respectful of everything around him.

"No. No, it's nothing. What did you call me for?" she said angrily.

"Are you—crying?" Carlos asked, incredulous, "Super-nurse is crying?"

"Shut up, Carlos," Clancy said as she walked back to the nurse's station just as the phone began ringing.

An hour passed before Lily emerged from the room with Ernest following dutifully behind her. Lily turned and took his hand in hers. He smiled as though this simple gesture implied that all was well. She spoke to him quietly and he nodded, his expression a question mark.

Clancy tried not to care. She tried to look away. But it was too late. Lily motioned to her from across the room. Clancy felt guilt shoot through her like lightening. Had Lily known that she'd been hiding in the shadows listening to their conversation? Feeling sheepish, she wove her way through roaming residents to Lily.

"Mother's not doing well," Lily said simply, "I know about her heart. I know about her medical problems. The hospital doctors told me not to expect her to be able..." Clancy waited. There was no question for her to answer. She studied Lily's face, noticing that it was still damp and swollen from crying. Instinctively her hand went up to her own face. She blotted under her eyes with her fingertips. Her skin was dry. She could appear professional.

"All I want to know is this," Lily leveled her gaze at Clancy. "The Alzheimer's—has it left my mother with anything? Is there anything? I mean, what does she know at this point?"

"In regards to what, exactly?" Clancy said. The question was too broad, too vague, and too unanswerable. Clancy watched Lily's eyes fill with tears.

"I mean does she know me at all? Do you think that when she calls me momma that she's only just forgotten my name?" Lily's eyes were wide and pleading.

"Of course she knows it's you. She still knows who she's talking to. She knows her own daughter. She just says momma because it's easier," Clancy used her most reassuring voice. Surprising even herself, she reached forward and gave Lily a quick hug. "She knows you. Your mother knows you. Of course she knows you. She does."

Moments later, after Lily had returned to Annabelle's room, Clancy remained where she was, watching her patients meander and drift. She imagined herself chiseling the essence of their existence out of a slab of soapstone or marble. She would do this. Maybe she would start the piece after work today.

"Liar," said a voice behind her. Clancy turned to see Carlos. He was shaking his head at her. "You know Annabelle doesn't know one person from the next anymore. Why did you tell her that? You fell all over that. You couldn't even shut up."

"How am I supposed to know what Annabelle knows? I have no real way of knowing what feelings mothers have for their daughter that go beyond words or recognition. It seems sort of, I don't know—spiritual or something," Clancy said softly without looking at him. "Leave it alone, Carlos. Haven't I told you a million times that I hate it when you try to be my conscience?"

"You're being incredibly metaphysical all of a sudden. It's weird. But interesting," he said teasingly, but his expression was full of concern. "Have you gone soft?"

"Don't you have work to do?" Clancy knew she had work to do, too. She shook off the emotions as though

they were raindrops on her lab coat and started back
down the hallway.

> *"Be like the bird*
> *That pausing in her flight*
> *Awhile on boughs too slight*
> *Feels them give way*
> *Beneath her and yet sings*
> *Knowing that she hath wings."*
> — *Victor Hugo*

CHAPTER 18

Lily

The grain elevators on the east side of Beau Lake, Minnesota cast long blue shadows across the dilapidated Petunia Street homes. The railroad track ran so close to the houses that it was a wonder they hadn't been shaken to bits years before. But the houses still stood. They'd been fine houses once. Two-story Victorian homes with elaborate lattice work and stained glass windows. Someone had painted them pastel pink, green and yellow in an attempt to salvage their essence. But the paint had become chipped and worn over time, leaving bare wood to show through like a skeleton. They had become two- and three-family dwellings, rented cheaply without leases. Older model cars parked in the gravel driveways added to the tone of disrepair. No one cared anymore. The passing trains would eventually wear the houses down to nubs on the dead end street, leaving the cars to rust into heaps of useless metal.

Canadian geese inhabited the other side of the road along the bank of a small nameless lake bordered by cottonwood trees. The geese landed every morning with a rush of wing beats and loud honking as they claimed the grain spilled from trucks traveling to and from the elevators. As the day wore on, the cackling geese sounded more and more like old ladies mocking the tattered homes. Stubborn houses that refused to be toppled by time and trains.

Just as the sun began to set on the small lake, Lily pulled her rental car alongside a giant fir tree on Petunia Street and stopped. She turned the ignition off and reclined her seat. The sky was beginning to bleed pink into blue. She looked up at the windows of 631 Petunia Street and saw the setting sun reflected in the glass. The curtains were partially drawn. There was no sign of life. She decided no one was home. There was nothing to do but wait. She pulled her jacket hood up over her head and folded her arms across her chest for warmth. Her breath came out in vapor puffs, causing the car windows to frost.

It was mid-May and still cold. One year had passed since Lily had brought her mother to Minnesota to find the red box. A year since her father had died unexpectedly.

She was still sleepy from the long drive from Texas to Minnesota. And there was the unbearable grief that had followed her like a predator after prey. Annabelle was gone. Her flawed heart had stopped beating. Her clouded brain had stopped destroying itself. Lily had sold her parent's Texas home. She had sold her Green Thumb Garden Shoppe. She'd said her final good-bye to her ex-fiancé. She had left hoping to erase the state of melancholy that engulfed her after Annabelle's death.

The deep blue of nightfall began to overtake the lavender sky. The temperature was dropping with the absence of daylight. The air was crisp and cold. Lily shivered. She rubbed her hands together and blew warm breath on them. The geese's honking and cackling became more hushed as though the approaching night had muffled them with a blanket.

By the time the old Chevy pick-up truck pulled into the driveway at 631 Petunia Street, one lone street light had buzzed on, casting a dim yellow light across the pastel houses. Lily watched the man as he opened the truck's door against a creaky protest of worn out hinges. Orange cigarette ashes flickered to the ground, followed by a puff of smoke and the man's hacking cough. He sat in the driver's seat for a long time looking up at the sky, his hand still on the door handle. Finally he dropped both feet to the ground, then swung around to retrieve a six pack of beer from the cab. He rubbed his eyes and then his neck, removed his baseball cap and tossed it into the truck. After another spasm of coughing, he slammed the door and stood beside the truck, gazing again at the sky, which was now pinpointed with tiny stars. He looked toward the quietly cackling geese and began again to rub the back of his neck. Lily sank deeper into her seat, praying he didn't see her there.

She watched as he fumbled with his keys, then opened the door and was swallowed up by the shabby darkened house. A whole five minutes passed before he switched on lights. Overhead lights. Bare bulbs hanging from the ceiling. His shadow loomed across each room he entered. Then, one by one the lights were switched off, replaced by a blue television screen light that filled the downstairs room. He didn't bother pulling the shade She could see him pop open a beer, light a cigarette, then sink into an overstuffed chair, plopping his feet onto the coffee table in front of him.

Lily watched him watching his television, sipping his beer, sucking in the smoke of his cigarette, stretching, rubbing his eyes and neck. Most likely, he would fall asleep there, waking up in time to return to his job at the hardware store the next day.

He was a handsome man. Long and lean with graying hair and dark eyes. He had a confidence in his gait that seemed to suggest he'd been someone important at one time. What had happened, Lily wondered. What could have happened to bring him here to this lonely house flanked by grain elevators, a nameless lake and cackling geese on a dead end road, drinking beer into the early hours of the morning? What would become of him? Was this all there would ever be for him? Someday would he be found dead in his overstuffed chair, beer in hand, an *I Love Lucy* rerun on the television screen?

Lily thought of Stanley, her father. She thought of his endless supply of books and his enthusiasm for outdoor adventure, his love of teaching. She thought of his unconditional love for Annabelle and his ability to hide her emotional flaws. Lily thought of his love for her, his daughter. A daughter who was never his biological child but was cherished even more because of it.

Stanley had planned to tell Lily this, but Annabelle refused. It had terrified Annabelle. As though by revealing this to her daughter, Lily would somehow turn criminal. Or worse. She could become insignificant. She might throw her life away. She might become the same as this man, her uncle Frankie, who sat sipping his beer, staring at his television in a ramshackle house on the east side of Beau Lake, Minnesota.

Lily had rehearsed what she might say to Frankie. She'd rehearsed what she would say the moment he opened his door. She'd practiced her introduction. Her parents were gone now, she'd finally tell him. I have no family. Your brother was my father. I just thought—

My mother killed your brother. I'm so sorry. She was so sorry. It's just that she came from such a violent, horrible home. It was her parents. They made my mother psychotic. They were disturbed people. Criminal, really. They'd murdered her older sister. My mother was only a child, but she was in the boat—she saw it happen. She had always been afraid. Afraid of everything, really. I just thought that maybe—

A full moon rose slowly from the depths of the blue night. The geese were silent now. The cold air had turned bitter as a north wind whipped around the grain elevators. Lily turned the key in the ignition. She pulled away from Petunia Street and did not look back.

By morning the wind had shifted, bringing warm air from the south. Lily pulled back cottage curtains, opening every window in the cabin, letting sunlight dance across the rooms. The south breeze swirled through the house, forcing out darkness. Forcing out old demons. Filling the house with new air that she would now own.

She made strong coffee and sat sipping it on the beach as she gazed out over the sparkling lake in front of her. The expanse of blue water was speckled with tiny white dots of sunlight. Like diamonds or pearls bobbing on the lake's surface, she thought. Just like tiny pearls.

Her mother's sister Hazel, only a teenager, and pregnant, was rowed out into the middle of this lake by Lily's grandparents. Maybe at this very spot. They'd commanded her to dive over the side of the boat and told her to swim back to shore. It was her punishment. But she never made it. It was too far. The water was too frigid. The authorities had ruled her drowning an accident. The entire event had dissipated within a short period of time. Except in the memory of Hazel's baby sister Annabelle who had also been in the boat. Watching, but not understanding. Not until years later when she would be frozen by the horror of it like suddenly being trapped in a bottomless nightmare.

Lily shuddered. She would think of this many times before the shock of it would finally numb her. But today, she would start over. She would go into town and find her childhood friend Tess at the Gray Dawn Café where they would eat breakfast together, discussing their hopes and dreams. She would see Will Larson, Sam and Teddy Olson and a whole new generation of townspeople who never knew of her grandparents living at Cattails End. A generation who had no knowledge of the illness that had gripped her grandmother, mother and perhaps someday, Lily herself. She would simply start over. She would redeem every wrong thing that had happened to her mother.

Thirty minutes later, the aroma of baking bread and freshly brewed coffee greeted Lily as she entered the Gray Dawn. She spotted Tess instantly. Teddy sat across from his mother in a booth at the back, facing the door. He broke into a wide grin and waved to Lily as she walked toward their table.

"Lily!" Tess jumped up and hugged her friend. "I didn't know you were going to be here yet. Why didn't you tell me? I thought you weren't going to come until after you sold your shop."

"I did sell it," Lily said as she slipped into the booth next to Teddy. She glanced around the café, noticing new paintings on the walls. "Is this your work?"

"Some of it." Teddy looked at the art work with mild interest. "It's old stuff, though. I'm having a one-man show in Minneapolis next month. All new paintings."

"Really? Wow!" Lily patted him on the shoulder, realizing suddenly that he wasn't a kid anymore. "Congratulations."

"Order something. You look skinny." Tess handed Lily a menu, quickly adding, "But you look good. Really good. So you're okay, then?"

"Great. I am absolutely great. What about you guys?" Lily noticed that the café was crowded with people she'd never seen before. "A lot of customers this morning. Is it because it's Saturday?"

"Snowbirds coming back from their homes in the south," Tess shrugged. "You know, tourist season for the lake starts around Memorial Day."

Lily did know this. She smiled inwardly thinking that she had once been considered a snowbird.

"Hey, I've gotta go," Teddy said, looking at his watch. "I'm supposed to start painting a mural at the library in Beau Lake this morning. Great seeing you again, Lily. Later."

The two women watched him dash away just as Will Larson strolled through the swinging doors that led from the kitchen. He saw Lily and waded through the tables of customers to greet her.

"How are you, Lily?" His welcoming smile quickly faded to somber empathy. "So sorry about your mom. Tough year for you. You okay?"

"Sure. Yeah, I'm good." Lily smiled up at him.

"That's good. How long are you going to be—" he started, but stopped abruptly when a customer called to him from another table. "Man, it's really busy in here this morning. Let me get the waitress to bring you some coffee and the muffins I just baked. And anything else you want. We'll talk later, okay?"

"Sure, okay." Lily watched him walk away, then turned to Tess. "The waitress?"

"I know. He has a waitress helping him now," Tess said. "Can you believe it? His café is getting really popular." She blotted her mouth with her napkin and pushed the plate away, holding her cup in the air to summon the matronly waitress who scuffled over to their booth with a coffee pot and a tray of muffins.

Lily took slow sips of her coffee, savoring the warmth of it. She felt the melancholy gloom that had been her constant companion for the past months begin to slip away.

"So you sold the shop? I cannot believe it," Tess said. Her blue eyes were wide and childlike just as they had always been. Her life had been grounded in this town since the day she was born. Everyone loved Tess. There was nothing not to love.

"I took another position," Lily said.

"Really? Where? What is it?" Tess asked. She was brushing tiny crumbs off the table onto the floor.

"Beau Lake. I'm going to be the new editor of the *Beau Lake Daily News*." Lily beamed. It was the perfect job for her. If only Annabelle could've known.

"No! Are you serious?" Tess shrieked, "This is so cool. So you're moving here for good? Is that even possible?"

"It's a fact," Lily laughed. She took Tess's outstretched hand from across the table and squeezed it. "It's the truth. I'm here now."

"This is such wonderful news. After all you've been through." Tess's expression became suddenly pensive. "Was it just awful, Lily? At the end? Did Annabelle still know you?'

"I don't know," Lily drifted into the memory of Annabelle's last days. "You remember Clancy—her nurse? She said Annabelle knew me, but I don't think so. And I'm not sure it mattered."

"Clancy? You mean that nurse you said was a red-haired witch?"

"Well, yes, but she was okay. Especially at the end."

"But Clancy should know, right?" Tess said encouragingly, "What about that doctor? Ernest. Was that his name? Is he still a patient there? He must miss Annabelle terribly."

"He's still there. He hasn't changed much." Lily felt a pang of guilt as though she'd left him behind purposefully. "The taxi driver, you know—Pearl, comes to see him regularly now. He really enjoys that."

"Oh. Well, that's good," Tess smiled briefly, "but what about Annabelle's dog? Did you bring him with you?"

"No. Caesar died in his sleep a few days after Mother passed away," Lily said, blowing lightly on her coffee. She remembered how she'd found the dog that morning, curled into his wicker dog bed, unmoving. She'd burst into tears, suddenly aware of her deep attachment to the old basset hound. Her mother had loved him so much. Lily had laid her head on his breathless body and sobbed for all the memories of his short dog life.

"Oh my god, that is so incredibly sad. I'm so sorry. How eerie that he died right after she did—as though he somehow knew. Or maybe her spirit came to get him." Tess shook her head thinking of this. Her eyes took on a whimsical glow.

"He was really old, Tess. I think he was just tired." Lily felt the old sorrow begin to well up inside her. She closed her eyes and took a deep breath, dismissing the topic.

"But what about that red box? What was in it? Did you ever look?" Tess leaned forward, resting her elbows on the table.

"Yes. There was nothing. You know, just some old insurance papers, nothing important." Lily began to stare at one of Teddy's paintings. It was the silhouette of a woman standing on a dock looking out at a storm brewing over the ice-crusted lake. The woman was wearing no shoes, just socks.

"I wonder why she was so determined to find it then," Tess said.

"Probably the Alzheimer's playing with her brain." Lily continued to stare at the painting, remembering the night before when she'd driven away from Frankie's house on Petunia Street. Remembering how she had returned to the cabin so chilled that her bones felt like ice deep inside her body. Had she been cold from the temperature or from the realization that things would never be the same again?

She'd built a roaring fire in the woodstove and sat beside it, holding the open red box in her lap. And one by one, she burned Annabelle's heartbreaking journals, her letters, and every photograph, keeping only the small locket with the photo of her Aunt Hazel whom she had never known.

"Yeah, you're right.   " Tess sounded unsure as she studied Lily's face but did not intrude.

"She called me 'momma,'" Lily said wistfully.

"Momma," Tess said. "She thought you were her mother?"

"I think so," Lily turned her gaze to rest on her friend.

"Oh, that's sad, Lily. I'm sorry."

"No, it's okay. It doesn't make me sad at all. Annabelle needed to feel that her own mother had come to care for her finally. It's really okay. Even if she didn't know it, she felt it. She could still feel love and redemption."

Tess said nothing. She didn't understand. Could not understand. Sympathy was etched into her face, making her look old and uncertain. Finally, she looked away.

Sunlight peered through the heavy cloud cover of morning, forcing its way through the window to their table, illuminating everything in its path. Lily thought of the poems and short stories she had written after Annabelle died. She knew now that she would tuck them into the empty red box until the day when they would either be published or stored away for someone else to find.

Lily had forgiven Annabelle. And for one clear instant in her sea of confusion, Annabelle had forgiven her own mother. It was as it should be.

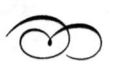

TO ORDER THIS BOOK

When Color Fades
a novel by C.J. Clark

If unavailable at your favorite bookstore,
we will fill your order promptly

—Postal Orders —

Carol Clark
www.cjclarkartist.com
E-mail: cjclark144@att.net

or

LangMarc Publishing
P.O. Box 90488 • Austin, Texas 78709-0488
Order online at www.langmarc.com
or call 1-800-864-1648
E-mail: langmarc@booksails.com

When Color Fades

(Paperback) U.S.A. $16.95 + $3 postage
Texas residents add 8.25% sales tax
Canada: $20.95 + postage